Cognitive Behavioral
Treatment of Insomnia

Michael L. Perlis, PhD
Sleep and Neurophysiology Research
  Laboratory
Behavioral Sleep Medicine Service
Department of Psychiatry
University of Rochester
Rochester, NY 14642
USA

Michael T. Smith, PhD
Department of Psychiatry and
  Behavioral Sciences
The Johns Hopkins University
Baltimore, MD 21287
USA

Carla Jungquist, MSN, FNP-C
Sleep and Neurophysiology Research
  Laboratory
Behavioral Sleep Medicine Service
Department of Psychiatry and School
  of Nursing
University of Rochester
Rochester, NY 14642
USA

Donn Posner, PhD
Department of Psychiatry and Human
  Behavior
Sleep Disorders Center of Lifespan
  Hospitals
Brown Medical School
Providence, RI 02912
USA

Library of Congress Control Number: 2005924097

ISBN 10: 0-387-22252-9   Printed on acid-free paper.
ISBN 13: 978-0387-22252-3

Printed in the United States of America.   (BS/MVY)

9 8 7 6 5 4 3 2 1   SPIN 10984222

springeronline.com

Cognitive Behavioral Treatment of Insomnia

A Session-by-Session Guide

Michael L. Perlis, PhD
Sleep and Neurophysiology Research Laboratory, Behavioral Sleep Medicine Service, Department of Psychiatry, University of Rochester, Rochester, New York, USA

Carla Jungquist, MSN, FNP-C
Sleep and Neurophysiology Research Laboratory, Behavioral Sleep Medicine Service, Department of Psychiatry and School of Nursing, University of Rochester, Rochester, NY, USA

Michael T. Smith, PhD
Department of Psychiatry and Behavioral Sciences, The Johns Hopkins University, Baltimore, Maryland, USA

Donn Posner, PhD
Department of Psychiatry and Human Behavior, Sleep Disorders Center of Lifespan Hospitals, Brown Medical School, Providence, Rhode Island, USA

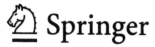 Springer

To our patients: Thank you for showing us so much we didn't know. . . . May we serve you as well.

To Leisha Smith and Cindy Phillips: Thank you for your support and hard work, especially in the closing months of this project. Your influx of energy turned out to be an essential "counterfatigue measure."

To my parents, Edie and Marvin Perlis: Thank you for your love and guidance.

To Wally, Dick, Donn, and Donna: Thank you for your mentorship.

Michael L. Perlis

Brian and Danielle: Thanks for so graciously sharing me with my career and for giving me inspiration to always improve myself.

Bob: I am the person I am because of you.

Carla Jungquist

To Michelle: You are in the trenches with me every day. I could not do it without you, and there is nobody I would rather have there with me. Thank you.

To Nolan and Hailey: Someday you will know how much each of you inspire me. I only hope that I do the same for you.

To my parents: I am graced to have you.

To Meaghan: You are the strongest and sweetest person I know. Thanks for being there.

Michael T. Smith

To Karen: You are my center. Without you I would surely be adrift. Thank you for being someone I can hold on to.

To Max: You bring so much joy and fun into my life. You are the best! Go Yanks!

Donn Posner

Foreword

The treatment of insomnia has reached a milestone. Cognitive Behavior Therapy (CBT) has achieved wide-spread scientific recognition as an effective treatment for a wide variety of insomnias. This approach is made up of a number of components, including initial assessments, the integration of validated cognitive behavioral treatment interventions for insomnia, and methods for helping to ensure that patients follow through with treatment instructions between sessions as well as after treatment has been completed. The manual provides a useful discussion of assessment techniques and the role of sleep diaries, actigraphy, and polysomnography in the treatment of insomnia.

While many behaviorally oriented clinicians have experience with at least one of the components that comprise CBT, too few have used this approach with its full complement of interventions in a systematic manner. This manual is a superb tool that clinicians can use to sharpen their skills to effectively treat insomnia. The authors' approach resonates with us in that they systematically integrate empirically validated components from the insomnia treatment literature, including stimulus control therapy, sleep restriction therapy, sleep hygiene education, and cognitive therapy into a state-of-the art treatment. The authors have not merely cobbled together a random set of techniques, but, rather, each component has been carefully selected and intergrated with the others. The authors have been in the forefront of those doing both clinical research and treatment for chronic insomnia. This manual reflects their collective experience and deep understanding of the challenges in helping patients with chronic insomnia improve their sleep.

Although, in general, manuals are most useful for beginners, this book has something for everyone. As seasoned clinicians, we found the weave of therapist–patient dialogues, treatment options, rationale, and skillful handling of potential patient resistance produced an insightful and thought provoking presentation that enlarged our understanding and appreciation of the subtlety of the clinical enterprise. There is much wisdom in this book.

One of the particularly useful features is the many sample dialogues between therapist and patient that provide examples of how components

of the treatment are introduced, how to provide the rationale for the treatment, how to answer questions that patients have, how to help ensure effective implementation, and how to prepare patients for anticipating problems and preventing relapse after treatment ends. The therapist in the dialogues is very effective. The treatment is conducted in a systematic manner, the bases for the therapeutic interventions are explained and metaphorically illustrated, and the therapist's manner engages the patient sufficiently to garner active collaboration. In addition to the nuts and bolts of what to do and when that is the mandate of a treatment manual, we believe there is much to be learned from modeling a therapeutic approach as is done here.

As many readers will know, the two of us are identified with the development and evaluation of single behavioral components in the treatment of insomnia—stimulus control therapy (RRB) and sleep restriction therapy (AJS). It has not been lost on us that our joint writing of this foreword symbolically represents the CBT approach to insomnia (i.e., a multicomponent approach that integrates diverse components to address the multiple determinants that result in chronic insomnia). The authors of this manual are quite savvy and have used even the opportunity of the foreword to make the point that single-component approaches do not serve all clinical patients equally well. We have patients to help and this manual does a superb job in presenting the straightforward and effective approach of CBT within the framework of the complexity that is the human condition.

Richard R. Bootzin, PhD
Professor of Psychology and Psychiatry
Director, Insomnia Program
Department of Psychology and Department of Psychiatry
University of Arizona
Tucson, Arizona

Arthur J. Spielman, PhD
Professor, Department of Psychology
The City College of the City University of New York
Associate Director, Center for Sleep Medicine
Weill Medical College, Cornell University
New York, New York

Preface

There is now an overwhelming preponderance of evidence that Cognitive Behavioral Therapy for Insomnia (CBT-I) is effective (1;2), as effective as sedative hypnotics during acute treatment (4–8 weeks) (3;4), and more effective in the long term (following treatment) (3). In general, CBT-I yields an average treatment effect of about 50% improvement, with large effect sizes that are reliably around 1.0 (1;2;4). Longitudinal studies provide good evidence of sustained treatment effects for Sleep Latency (SL) and Wake After Sleep Onset (WASO) and more substantial improvement with time for Total Sleep Time (TST) (1) (2;5).

Given that CBT-I has been rigorously empirically validated, it is now time to make available a treatment manual that provides a precise guide to treatment. This manual is intended to fill this need and to provide a level of description that is sufficiently articulated as to allow:

- Clinicians from other fields and clinical students to begin the process of learning to provide empirically validated CBT-I,
- Practicing behavioral sleep medicine clinicians information that may help to refine and/or expand their CBT-I skills, and
- Clinical trialists to deliver standardized therapy.

For the first group of would-be "end users," we strongly suggest that training in this area works best using an apprenticeship model and accordingly recommend that a series of mentored experiences be used to augment the materials presented in this manual. For trainees within clinical sleep medicine programs, arranging for mentorship may be easily accomplished. For community-based clinicians, arranging for mentorship may be more challenging, but can be accomplished by peer supervision and/or telephone consultation with established behavioral sleep medicine specialists.

This manual has seven sections. The seven sections are as follows:

- The definition of insomnia,
- A brief review of the conceptual framework for treatment,
- An overview of the components of therapy,
- A session-by-session guide,
- An extended dialogues section,
- A case example: Assessment and Eligibility for CBT-I & Sample Documentation,
- Appendices.

While the intent of the first two chapters is clear from their titles, the purpose of the five remaining chapters requires some explanation. The *components of therapy* chapter reviews the primary therapeutic modalities, indicates what patients are appropriate for CBT-I, makes recommendations regarding clinician credentials, discusses what constitutes the ideal clinic setting, and suggests a useful approach to charting. The *session-by-session* chapter delineates the tasks and goals for each session and provides some background information and dialogue examples of how treatment is delivered. The dialogues are not intended to be scripts for the clinician to memorize, but simply concrete examples of how therapy is conducted. The *extended dialogues* section provides a series of examples of questions that patients tend to raise and provides sample responses. The *case example* chapter applies our algorithm to demonstrate whether a particular patient is a candidate for CBT-I. We also provide an example of session-by- session notes that follow the patient through a course of treatment, along with treatment graphs and an example of a summary letter to the patient's primary care physician. The *appendices* provide copies of some instruments that may be of use (e.g., intake questionnaires, sleep diaries, examples of chart graphs, etc.).

The organizing principles for the manual are "Who is appropriate for CBT-I?" and "What does one need to know to set up a behavioral sleep medicine service that is prepared to deliver empirically validated, data-driven and data-yielding treatment?" With respect to the issue of "who is appropriate," the approach used in this manual is not diagnosis-based but rather indication-based. That is, we present an algorhithmic approach to the decision process. One is eligible for treatment not because the person meets the criteria for certain diagnoses, but rather because the symptoms appear to be maintained by factors that are targeted by, and amenable to, CBT-I. This is not to suggest that diagnosis is irrelevant. The diagnostic process allows the clinician to determine what other factors and disease issues require treatment beyond CBT-I or whether CBT-I is contraindicated.

One final preliminary note: This manual is intended to be narrowly focused on the provision of CBT-I. For a more expansive review of Sleep Medicine and Behavioral Sleep Medicine, the reader is referred to the following texts: Principles & Practice of Sleep Medicine. Eds. Kryger, Roth & Dement. Fourth Edition. W.B. Saunders Co. Philadelphia. 2005; Sleep Disorders Medicine. Second Ed. Chokroverty. Butterworth-Heinemann. Boston. 1999; Treating Sleep Disorders: The Principles & Practice of Behavioral Sleep Medicine. Eds. Perlis & Lichstein. Wiley & Sons. 2003; and Insomnia: A Clinician's Guide to Assessment and Treatment Eds. Morin & Espie. Plenum Pub Corp. 2003.

Michael L. Perlis, PhD
Carla Jungquist, MSN, FNP-C
Michael T. Smith, PhD
Donn Posner, PhD

Acknowledgments

Over the course of this project we have been fortunate to have the ability to seek input from many of the people who are active in the nascent field of Behavioral Sleep Medicine. Accordingly, we want to acknowledge and thank the following individuals for sharing their time and perspectives.

Richard Bootzin, University of Arizona
Daniel Buysse, University of Pittsburgh

Jack Edinger, Duke University
Ken Lichstein, University of Alabama
Art Spielman, City College of New York
Edward Stepanski, Rush-Presbyterian

Colin Espie, University of Glasgow
Charles Morin, Laval University

Celyne Bastien, Laval University
Allison Harvey, University of California at Berkeley

Sara Matteson, University of Rochester Sleep and Neurophysiology Research Laboratory

Wilfred R. Pigeon, University of Rochester Sleep and Neurophysiology Research Laboratory

Michael L. Perlis, PhD
Carla Jungquist, MSN, FNP-C
Michael T. Smith, PhD
Donn Posner, PhD

About the Authors

Michael L. Perlis, PhD
Dr. Perlis is an Associate Professor of Psychiatry and URMC Neurosciences Program at the University of Rochester. He is also the Director of the UR Sleep Research Laboratory and Director of the UR Behavioral Sleep Medicine Service. His clinical expertise is in the area of Behavioral Sleep Medicine. His research interests include sleep in psychiatric disorders and neurocognitive phenomena in insomnia, the mechanisms of action for CBT-I and of sedative hypnotics, and the development of alternative treatments for insomnia. He is the Sr. Editor for the first text book for the field of Behavioral Sleep Medicine, he is on the editorial board for the Journal of Behavioral Sleep Medicine, and he was a founding member of the American Academy of Sleep Medicine's committee for Behavioral Sleep Medicine.

Carla Jungquist, MSN, FNP-C
Ms. Jungquist is a Family Nurse Practitioner who specializes in pain and sleep. She works as a clinician at the UR Behavioral Sleep Medicine Service. She also serves as medical consultant for the University of Rochester Sleep Research Laboratory, and is a co-principal-investigator on a NIH funded study to evaluate Cognitive Behavioral Therapy for Insomnia in Chronic Pain Patients. She is a member of the Board of Directors for the Association of Pain Management Nurses and is a Doctoral Candidate at the University of Rochester School of Nursing.

Michael T. Smith, PhD
Dr. Smith is Assistant Professor of Psychiatry and Behavioral Sciences at Johns Hopkins University School of Medicine. He is a licensed clinical psychologist and is certified in Behavioral Sleep Medicine by the American Academy of Sleep Medicine. Dr. Smith conducts clinical research and practices at the Johns Hopkins Behavioral Medicine Research Laboratory and Clinic. His research specializes in the neurobehavioral causes and conse-

quences of insomnia and sleep deprivation, particularly as it occurs in chronic pain conditions.

Donn Posner, PhD

Dr. Posner is a Clinical Assistant Professor of Psychiatry and Human Behavior at the Brown Medical School. He is also the Director of the Behavioral Sleep Medicine Program for the Sleep Disorders Center of Lifespan Hospitals in Providence Rhode Island. He has been actively engaged in the treatment of sleep-disordered patients for the past sixteen years. For eleven of those years he has served as the lead supervisor and mentor for a sleep medicine rotation in the behavioral medicine track of the Brown Clinical Psychology Internship. He is a member of the American Academy of Sleep Medicine and recently became one of the first certified behavioral sleep medicine specialists recognized by that group.

Contents

Foreword *by Richard R. Bootzin and Arthur J. Spielman* vii

Preface ix

Acknowledgments xi

About the Authors xiii

Featured Dialogues xvii

1 The Definition of Insomnia 1

2 The Conceptual Framework for CBT-I 7

3 The Components of Therapy 12

4 CBT-I Session by Session 34

5 CBT-I Example Dialogues for Patient Questions and Challenges 105

6 A Case Example 121

References 142

Glossary 148

Appendices 159
1 The Calculation of Sleep Efficiency 161
2 Example of Clinic Brochure 163
3 Example of Treatment Graphs 165
4A Medical History Checklist 166

4B Medical Symptom Checklist 167
4C The Sleep Disorders Symptom Checklist 168
4D Sleep Environment Checklist 170
4E Motivation for Change Index 171
5   Single Day Sleep Diary 172
6   "Week at a Glance" Sleep Diary 174

Index   175

Featured Dialogues

Dialogue 1   Patient Description of Insomnia   7
Dialogue 2   Therapist Introduces Self to Patient   35
Dialogue 3   Presentation of Treatment Options   43
Dialogue 4   Should I Continue with My Current Medications
             While in Treatment?   46
Dialogue 5   Why Can't I Start Treatment Immediately?   47
Dialogue 6   Setting Expectations for Weekly Agenda   48
Dialogue 7   Discussion of the "Mismatch" Between TIB
             and TST....................................   51
Dialogue 8   Discussion of Predisposing, Precipitating, and
             Perpetuating Factors   52
Dialogue 9   Setting up Sleep Restriction and Stimulus
             Control   55
Dialogue 10 "Why Can't I at Least Rest in Bed?"   57
Dialogue 11 Confirming Patient's Understanding of The
             "To Do" List   59
Dialogue 12 What Happens If I Enjoy Staying Up Too Much? ..   61
Dialogue 13 Confirming TST Is Calculated and Not Estimated ..   64
Dialogue 14 Dealing with Noncompliance Using Cognitive
             Restructuring   67
Dialogue 15 What ... I Have to Restrict Myself More?   69
Dialogue 16 Sleep Hygiene #1: Homeostat, Wake Time, and
             Exercise   71
Dialogue 17 Sleep Hygiene #2: Exercise Alternatives and
             Bedroom Environment   73
Dialogue 18 Sleep Hygiene #3: Regular Meals, Fluid Restriction,
             and Caffeine   75
Dialogue 19 Sleep Hygiene #4: Alcohol and Nicotine   76
Dialogue 20 Sleep Hygiene #5: Don't Take Problems to Bed   78
Dialogue 21 Sleep Hygiene #6: Don't Try to Fall Asleep   80
Dialogue 22 Sleep Hygiene #7: Clock Watching and Naps   80
Dialogue 23 Discussion of Sleep State Misperception   85

Dialogue 24   Setting the Stage for Cognitive Restructuring   91
Dialogue 25   Calculating How Long the Patient Has Had
              Insomnia (in Days)   92
Dialogue 26   Identify and Record Catastrophic Thoughts   93
Dialogue 27   Assess the Patient's Probability Estimates   94
Dialogue 28   Determine the Actual Frequency of the Anticipated
              Catastrophes   94
Dialogue 29   Mismatch Between the Patient's Estimates and
              the Probability of Catastrophic Outcomes   95
Dialogue 30   Create a Countering Mantra to the Catastrophic
              Thoughts   96
Dialogue 31   What Happens If I Stop Sleeping Again?   102
Dialogue 32   I'm Having Trouble Filling Out the Sleep
              Diaries   105
Dialogue 33   Why Do I Have to Fill Out Sleep Diaries?   107
Dialogue 34   Shouldn't We Use Fancy Equipment to
              Measure My Sleep?   107
Dialogue 35   I Can't Seem to Remember to Fill Out My
              Diary   109
Dialogue 36   I'm Really Nervous About Stopping My Sleeping
              Pills   110
Dialogue 37   I Tried But Couldn't Stop Taking My Sleeping
              Pills   112
Dialogue 38   If I Don't Get to Sleep, How Am I Going to
              Function?   113
Dialogue 39   No, Really, There Have Been Times When I Haven't
              Functioned   114
Dialogue 40   I've Already Tried Behavioral Stuff and It Doesn't
              Work   116
Dialogue 41   There Is No Way I Can Stay Up That Late!   118

1
The Definition of Insomnia

In the early 1980s, as the sleep medicine movement was just gathering steam, there was perhaps no rallying cry as popular as "insomnia is a symptom, not a disorder." Presumably, this position was adopted because it was genuinely believed that the polysomnographic (PSG) study of sleep was destined to reveal all the underlying pathologies that give rise to the "symptoms" of not only insomnia but fatigue and sleepiness as well. After more than two decades of sleep research and sleep medicine, it is interesting to find that "all things old are new again": Insomnia is once again considered a distinct nosological entity. Below are the three primary definitions for insomnia, followed by some discussion regarding issues pertaining to chronicity, frequency and severity. This information is provided so that the reader can (1) have a firm grounding in "how insomnia is defined," and (2) can appreciate some of the difficulties associated with a diagnosis based approach to the problem of insomnia.

The Three Most Common Definitions of Insomnia

Insomnia

The World Health Organization defines insomnia as a problem initiating and/or maintaining sleep or the complaint of nonrestorative sleep that occurs on at least three nights a week and is associated with daytime distress or impairment (6).

Primary Insomnia

The term "primary insomnia," which is adopted by the American Psychiatric Association's diagnostic nomenclature (DSM-IV) (7)), is used to distinguish insomnia that is considered to be a distinct diagnostic entity from insomnia that is a symptom of an underlying medical and/or psychiatric condition. The American Psychiatric Association specifies a duration

criteria of one month and stipulates that the diagnosis be made when the predominant complaint is difficulty initiating or maintaining sleep or non-restorative sleep. In either case, the complaint must be associated with significant distress and daytime impairment, and must not be the result of other medical, psychiatric, or sleep disorders.

Psychophysiologic Insomnia

Within the American Academy of Sleep Medicine's nosology (the International Classification of Sleep Disorders-Revised [ICSD-R] (8)), primary insomnia is referred to as "psychophysiologic insomnia." The ICSD-R definition is more directly tied to the etiologic underpinnings of the disorder. The advantage of describing the disorder with this term is that it suggests how insomnia is initiated and maintained. Psychophysiologic insomnia is described as "a disorder of somatized tension and learned sleep-preventing associations that results in a complaint of insomnia and associated decreased functioning during wakefulness" (8). "Somatized tension" refers to either the patient's subjective sense of, or objective measures of, somatic hyperarousal while attempting to sleep. Somatic arousal is characterized by peripheral nervous system activity which is commonly marked by increased muscle tension, rapid heart rate, sweating, and so on. "Learned sleep-preventing associations" refers to the pattern of pre-sleep arousal that appears to be classically conditioned to the bedroom environment, where intrusive presleep cognitions, racing thoughts, and rumination are often taken as indicators of presleep arousal.

Interestingly, none of the nosologies formally embrace the older descriptive clinical characterizations of insomnia as initial, middle and terminal. *Initial Insomnia*, also referred to as "early," or "sleep-onset" insomnia, describes when the patient has trouble falling asleep. *Middle Insomnia*, also referred to as "sleep-maintenance" insomnia, describes when the patient has trouble with frequent or prolonged awakenings. *Terminal Insomnia*, also referred to as "late," or "early morning awakening" insomnia, describes when the patient awakens earlier than desired and is unable to fall back asleep. The fact that these terms do not constitute modern parlance should not keep the clinician from using the terms descriptively.

Disease Characteristics (Duration and Severity)

Apart from presenting a specific definition of the disorder/disease entity, there is the need to qualify the duration and severity of the defined illness. Typically, duration is framed dichotomously in terms of whether the illness is acute or chronic. Severity is, more often than not, defined solely in terms of frequency of complaint.

Duration of Illness

Insomnia lasting less than one month is generally considered "acute" and is often associated with clearly defined precipitants such as stress, acute pain, or substance abuse. Insomnia is characterized as being chronic when symptoms persist unabated for a duration of at least one month, and more typically for durations of time that are six months or greater. Please note that these cutoffs are relatively arbitrary and correspond to traditional medical definitions of what constitutes short and long periods of time. At present, no studies use risk models to evaluate the natural course of insomnia. Thus, there is no way of definitively defining "chronicity" in terms which are related to when the disorder becomes severe, persistent, and (for want of a better expression) "self-perpetuating."

One clinical cue for differentiating between acute and chronic insomnia resides in the way patients characterize their complaint. When patients stop causally linking their insomnia to its precipitant and instead indicate that their sleep problems seem "to have a life of their own," this change in presentation may (1) serve to define the "cut point" between the acute and chronic phases of the disorder and (2) suggest when CBT-I should be indicated.

Severity of Illness

Typically, severity is defined in terms of both symptom frequency and intensity. Both domains may be applied to insomnia, although—as noted—only symptom frequency tends to be embraced as a relevant diagnostic consideration.

Frequency

There is no fixed benchmark for what constitutes "frequent" symptoms. Most clinical researchers require that patients experience sleep problems on three or more nights per week. This cutoff may have more to do with increasing the odds of studying the occurrence of the disorder in laboratory than an inherent belief that less than three nights per week is "normal."

The more important issue here is that defining "severity" in terms of "frequency of symptoms" tacitly acknowledges that (1) insomnia symptoms typically do not occur every night and (2) the more frequent the symptom, the more severe the disorder. While the latter seems like a tautology, and for all diseases, this is especially important for how one thinks about insomnia. If the insomnia is more episodic, the occurrence of symptoms may be less related to the factors that are thought to be responsible for Primary Insomnia and more related to social, environmental, and/or circadian variables. Thus, it may be the case that traditional CBT-I may not be indicated for less severe insomnia (less frequent). Instead, this form of the disorder

may be best managed by identifying the variables that produce the insomnia on an intermittent basis and by providing a form of treatment which directly targets the idiosyncratic factors.

Intensity

No formal diagnostic criteria exist for what constitutes "severe" within this domain. Most clinical researchers consider 30 or more minutes to fall asleep and/or 30 or more minutes of wakefulness after sleep onset to represent the threshold between normal and abnormal sleep. Recent work by Lichstein and colleagues, however, suggests that this criteria should be set at "greater than 30 minutes," as this definition is better related to the occurrence of complaint in population studies (9). While this may seem an academic distinction, the finding speaks to the issue of what is considered normal or tolerable in our culture and what is abnormal. Moreover, the lower limit for what constitutes "severe" (i.e., 30 minutes) also may alert us to instances where there is a subjective complaint in the absence of generally accepted standards for what constitutes a sleep disturbance. For example, a patient who complains of sleep onset problems but reliably reports 15 minute sleep latencies. In these, albeit rare cases, failing to meet the standard may suggest to the clinician that some intervention other than CBT-I is indicated.

With respect to how much sleep is "normal," many investigators are reluctant to fix a value for this parameter. Of the investigators that are inclined to define "what is too little sleep," most set the cutoff at 6.0 or 6.5 hours per night. The reluctance to establish total sleep time parameters is due, in part, to the difficulty in establishing precisely what is abnormal. Representing what is pathological with a single number is too confounded by factors like age, prior sleep, and the individual's basal level of sleep need. The lack of an established total sleep time cutoff is also related to the possibility that profound sleep initiation or maintenance problems may occur in the absence of sleep loss. For example, the patient who regularly takes two hours to fall asleep and extends their sleep opportunity by two or more hours may not suffer any sleep loss and will have total sleep times that are, by any yard stick, normal.

This is an important distinction because it is often assumed that insomnia is synonymous with sleep deprivation and that it is sleep loss that mediates the daytime sequelae of the disorder. While it is certainly the case that daytime symptoms might be explained by chronic sleep loss, they need not be ascribable only to lack of sleep, or for that matter to sleep continuity*

---

* Sleep Continuity: Refers to the speed with which sleep is initiated and the degree to which sleep is consolidated. The five variables used to define sleep continuity are Sleep Latency (SL), Frequency of Nocturnal Awakenings (FNA), Wake After Sleep Onset (WASO) time, Total Sleep Time (TST) and Sleep Efficiency (SE%). See Glossary for further definitions of these terms.

disturbance. Instead, the quality of sleep obtained by patients with insomnia may also substantially contribute to cognitive and somatic complaints and daytime fatigue. For example, it has been shown that patients with insomnia reliably exhibit sleep micro-architectural disturbances such as enhanced high frequency EEG activity during NREM sleep (10–14). This type of activity, which appears to be independent from sleep continuity and architecture parameters, has been shown to be correlated with patient perceptions about their sleep quality and quantity (10;15;16).

Commonalities and Problems with Current Definitions

All of the above definitions show a degree of consistency, both in terms of what "is" and "is not" delineated. Common to all is that (1) insomnia is defined as a subjective complaint, (2) patients must report compromised daytime functioning, (3) there are no specific criteria for how much wakefulness is considered pathologic (prior to desired sleep onset or during the night), and (4) there are no criteria for how little total sleep must be obtained to fall outside the normal range. The latter two of these issues have already been explicated above. The former two require further discussion.

Insomnia as a Subjective Complaint

Defining insomnia as a subjective complaint without requiring objective verification of signs and symptoms has advantages and disadvantages. The advantage of having subjective criteria is that it recognizes the primacy of the patient's experience of distress or disease. That is, ultimately patients seek, comply with, and discontinue treatment based on their perception of wellness. The disadvantage is that such measures, when used alone, do not allow for a complete characterization of either the patient's condition or the disorder in general.

Insomnia and Daytime Impairment

The reason that daytime complaints are required for diagnosis is that in the absence of such complaints, it is possible that the phenomena of "short sleep" may be misidentified (by the clinician and/or patient) as insomnia. Frequent complaints associated with insomnia include fatigue, irritability, problems with attention and concentration, and distress directly related to the inability to initiate and/or maintain sleep.

Finally, two of the clinical nosologies (DSM-IV and the WHO definitions) allow for the complaint of nonrestorative sleep, in the absence of problems initiating or maintaining sleep, to be classified as "insomnia." Presumably, the rationale for this is that shallow non-restorative sleep is "not good sleep," therefore it is "not sleep," which is technically what the term in-

somnia means. While this may also seem an academic issue, this allowance substantially thins the diagnostic boundary between insomnia and the other intrinsic sleep disorders. For example, patients with obstructive sleep apnea and period leg movement disorder typically do not have problems initiating or maintaining sleep. In fact, their chief complaints are of excessive daytime sleepiness and nonrestorative sleep. Allowing nonrestorative sleep, in the absence of problems initiating or maintaining sleep, to be classified as "insomnia" blurs the diagnostic distinction between these clinical entities.

Concluding Comment

We are fortunate to have several nosologies that recognize insomnia as an independent or primary disorder. The various classification systems provide us the wherewithal to differentiate types of insomnia by both the presenting complaint and the factors that are thought to precipitate or perpetuate the illness. Perhaps what remains to be accomplished, from a definitional point of view, is for scholars and scientists to complete the characterization of this important disorder by providing for the formulation of a definition which formally lays out the research diagnostic criteria for insomnia. While this may not be essential for (in general) clinical practice or (in specific) for the determination of when CBT-I is indicated, a formal and complete definition will allow clinical researchers to conduct more productive investigations when the entity under study may be evaluated in its "chemically pure" form.

2
The Conceptual Framework for CBT-I

While nearly everyone refers to the nonpharmacologic treatment of insomnia as "cognitive behavioral therapy," the guiding perspective and principles that govern treatment (and in fact the primary treatments themselves) are behavioral.

The Behavioral Model of Insomnia, put forward by Spielman and Colleagues in 1987 (17), is the first, most articulated, and most widely cited theory regarding the etiology of chronic insomnia. The perspective provides a powerful point of view: one which is inclusive and allows for explanation, prediction and control. At the heart of the behavioral model is a diathesis-stress perspective which, by taking into account behavioral factors, allows one to (1) conceptualize how acute insomnia develops into a chronic condition and (2) conceive of what factors should be targeted for treatment. A schematic representation of the model is presented in Figure 2.1.

In brief, this three factor diathesis-stress model posits that insomnia occurs acutely in relation to both predisposing and precipitating factors and that the chronic form of the disorder is maintained by maladaptive coping behaviors (perpetuating factors). Thus, an individual may be prone to insomnia due to trait characteristics, experiences acute episodes because of precipitating factors, and suffer from a chronic form of the disorder because of behavioral factors. Interestingly, patients often describe their insomnia in precisely these terms.

Dialogue #1: Patient Description of Insomnia

Patient: I started having trouble sleeping three months ago when I had a job interview. I've always been high-strung and a bit of a worrier, but the stress of that interview really did me in. What I don't understand is that I got the job and things have been great ever since, but I still can't sleep. Its as if the insomnia has a life of its own.

Predisposing factors extend across the entire biopsychosocial spectrum. Biological factors include hyperarousal/hyperreactivity and/or an inher-

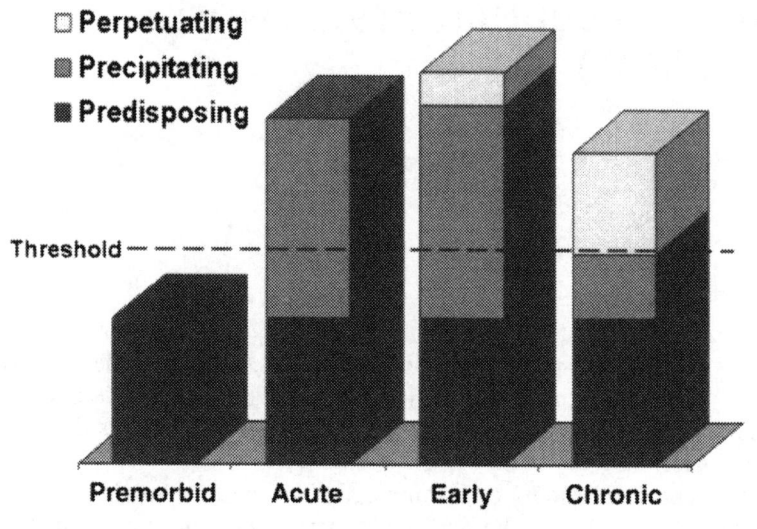

FIGURE 2.1. Nature of insomnia over time (Three-factor model from Spielman 1987).

ently weak sleep generating system. Psychological factors include worry or the tendency to be excessively ruminative. Social factors, although rarely a focus at the theoretical level, include such things as the bed partner keeping an incompatible sleep schedule or social/vocational pressures to sleep according to nonpreferred sleep schedule.

Precipitating factors are acute occurrences that interact with the patient's predisposition for insomnia to produce transient sleep initiation and/or maintenance problems. As with the Predisposing factors, the factors which precipitate acute insomnia also span the biopsychosocial spectrum. Biological factors include medical illness and injury, where these may either directly or indirectly give rise to insomnia. Psychological factors include acute stress reactions and/or the onset of psychiatric illness. Social factors include changes in the patient's social environment that require an acute shift in, or disrupt, one's preferred sleep phase (e.g., the need to provide infant care during the night).

Perpetuating factors refer to the variety of maladaptive strategies that individuals adopt in the face of transient insomnia in the attempt to get more sleep. Research and treatment have focused on two in particular: excessive time in bed and the increase in non-sleep related behaviors occurring in the bedroom. Spielman's three factor model tends to focus on the former: excessive time in bed. This refers to the tendency of patients with insomnia to go to bed earlier, get out of bed later, and/or nap. Such changes are enacted in order to increase the opportunity to get more sleep. These behaviors, however, lead to mismatch between sleep opportunity and

sleep ability. The greater the mismatch the more likely it is that the individual will spend prolonged periods of time awake during the given sleep period.

While not formally embraced within the Spielman model, the second of the maladaptive strategies is also considered perpetuating factor (the increase in non-sleep related behaviors occurring in the bedroom). This is thought to produce stimulus dyscontrol (a reduced likelihood that bed/bedroom-related stimuli will elicit a singular response given that such stimuli are paired with a wide array of behaviors). This concept is central to Bootzin's Stimulus Control perspective on insomnia (18).

The power of the behavioral model is that the therapeutic implications are clear. If chronic insomnia occurs primarily in relation to perpetuating factors, then the focus of behavioral treatment should be to eliminate the maladaptive behaviors that perpetuate the illness. That is, the focus of behavior therapy should be to control how much time is spent in bed (match sleep opportunity to sleep ability) and to prevent non-sleep behaviors from occurring in the bedroom. These are of course, the central components of Sleep Restriction (19) and Stimulus Control Therapy (18).

Finally, it is interesting to note that while the behavioral perspective allows for the concept of conditioned arousal, neither the Spielman Model nor Bootzin's Stimulus Control Perspective embrace the concept. Both, it seems to us, focus on the instrumental side of the behavioral equation; on the behaviors that maintain insomnia. In the case of sleep restriction, it is the behavior of increasing time in bed that leads to the mismatch between sleep opportunity and sleep ability. In the case of stimulus control, it is the nonsleep related behaviors that are engaged in within the sleep environment that weaken the association between sleep related cues and sleep. Neither perspective, in their original formulations, directly suggests that *being awake in bed sets the stage for a classical conditioning phenomena.* The repeated pairing of sleep related cues with wakefulness and/or arousal allows for the possibility that, in chronic insomnia, sleep related cues elicit arousal responses, and do so in the absence of (or in addition to) the other factors that maintain insomnia as a chronic illness.

It may well be the case that conditioned arousal is a final common factor or pathway for chronic insomnia. Put differently, the mismatch between sleep opportunity and sleep ability and poor stimulus control may perpetuate insomnia but only do so on a contingent basis. If the maladaptive behaviors occur, there is insomnia. If the maladaptive behaviors are modified or blocked, there is no insomnia. If, however, the contingency is protracted, there is the opportunity for a classical conditioning effect: conditioned arousal. This factor may perpetuate insomnia non-contingently and contribute to the disorder's apparently self perpetuating nature. If one takes into account the possibility that Chronic Insomnia may also involve a classical conditioning effect, this allows us a way to understand two of the most reliable findings from the treatment outcome literature. First, CBT-I

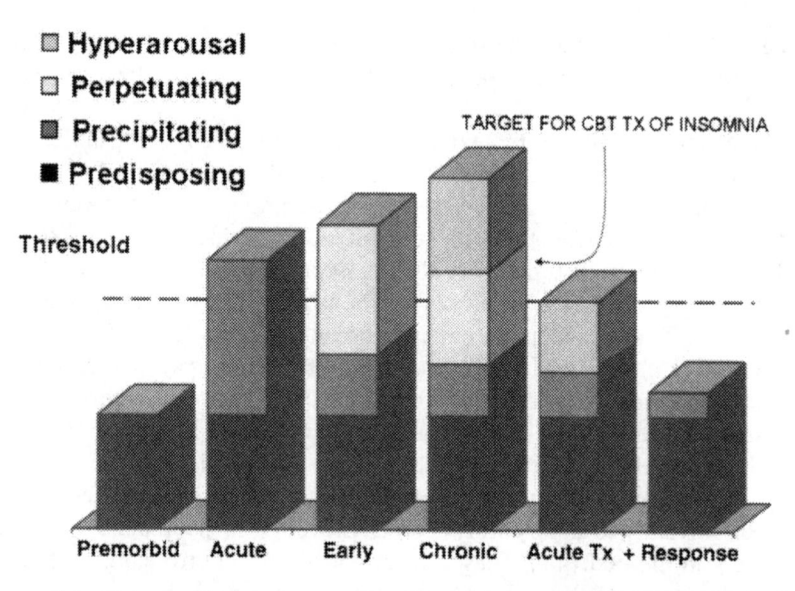

FIGURE 2.2. Nature of insomnia over time (four-factor model). As evident in Figure 2.1, the traditional Spielman Model does not extend to what occurs with treatment. The model is usually represented as ending with the "chronic phase." The "Acute Tx" and "+ Response" intervals are included here so that the reader may appreciate that (1) CBT-I eliminates the perpetuating factors and in so doing produces about 50% change and (2) the continued improvement over time may be the result of the counter-conditioning of hyperarousal (From Spielman 1987).

reliably produces about a 50% reduction in symptoms during the acute treatment phase* (e.g., 3;4). If only the traditional behavioral factors are responsible for chronic insomnia, one has to wonder why there is not a complete response to treatment. Second, following CBT-I patients continue to exhibit improvement over follow up periods as long as 12 months (e.g., 3;5). If only the traditional behavioral factors are responsible for chronic insomnia, one has to wonder why improvements occur beyond the acute treatment phase. If one allows for the possibility of conditioned arousal, then it may be that these effects occur as the conditioned arousal component abates with time (i.e., the repeated pairing of sleep related cues with sleep extinguishes the conditioned arousal). Thus, one can reasonably posit that classical conditioning or conditioned arousal is a factor in chronic insomnia and is appropriately subsumed under the Behavioral Perspective. To allow for a representation of this possibility, a version of the four factor

---

* The average 50% change from pre to post treatment applies to the combination of the symptoms that correspond to the patients presenting complaints "Can't fall asleep" (sleep latency 43% change) and "can't stay asleep" (wake after sleep onset 55%).

schematic is provided in Figure 2.2 which provides for this additional component.

Please note that while such a model as is presented in Figure 2.2 is plausible and well matched to the Behavioral perspective, there are a host of alternative explanations. It may be that with partial improvement (1) patients become more adherent with good maintenance strategies, (2) patients worry less as the problem becomes less frequent/severe, and (3) the stage is set for neurohormonal or functional brain changes that allow for continued recovery, and so on.

3
The Components of Therapy

What Are the Primary Components of Therapy?

This chapter briefly describes each of the first- and second-line treatments for insomnia. Elaborated explanations and specific instructions are provided in the portion of this manual dedicated to "session-by-session" information. The most common cognitive–behavioral therapies for chronic insomnia are: stimulus control, sleep restriction, sleep hygiene, relaxation training, and cognitive therapy. Typically, therapy includes three or more of the above components.

First-Line Interventions

What constitutes "first-line" is somewhat a matter of debate (21;22). Most clinical practices and clinical trials protocols adopt a multicomponent approach to treatment; where the components are usually stimulus control and/or sleep restriction therapy along with sleep hygiene instructions.

Stimulus Control Therapy (SCT)

This treatment modality is recommended for both sleep initiation and maintenance problems (18;23). The therapy is considered, according to the American Academy of Sleep Medicine (21), to be *the* first-line behavioral treatment for chronic insomnia. This is the case because this intervention has been assessed extensively as a monotherapy and has been found to reliably produce good clinical results.

Stimulus control instructions limit the amount of time one may spend in the bedroom while awake and the kind of behaviors one may engage in while in the bed/bedroom. These limitations are intended to strengthen the association between the bed/bedroom/bedtime with rapid, well-consolidated sleep. Typical instructions include: (1) lie down intending to go to sleep only when sleepy, (2) avoid any behavior in the bed or bedroom other

than sleep or sexual activity, (3) leave the bedroom if awake for more than 15 minutes, and (4) return to the bed only when sleepy. Items 3 and 4 are repeated as needed. Finally, keep a fixed wake time seven days a week, irrespective of the amount of sleep obtained. Some clinicians, in an effort to prevent "clock-watching" behavior, encourage patients to leave the bedroom as soon as they feel "clearly awake" or experience annoyance and irritation over the fact that they are awake.

As originally conceived of by Bootzin and colleagues in the early 1970s (18), this intervention is a direct application of a behavioral principle to the problem of insomnia. "Stimulus control" as a concept (versus a treatment modality) pertains to the idea that one stimulus may elicit many responses, depending on the conditioning history. A simple conditioning history wherein the stimulus is always paired with a single response yields a high probability that the stimulus will yield only one response. A complex conditioning history wherein the stimulus is paired with a variety of responses yields a low probability that the stimulus will yield only one response. As applied to the problem of insomnia, the idea is that the normal cues that are associated with sleep (bed, bedroom, bedtime, etc.) are too frequently paired with responses other than sleep. That is, in an effort to cope with the insomnia, the patient spends too much time in the bed/bedroom awake and engaging in behaviors other than sleep.

These coping behaviors appear to the patient to be both reasonable and reasonably successful. With respect to the latter, the strategies appear to work "some of the time." With respect to the former, "staying in bed when awake" allows for the opportunity to get more sleep and has the virtue of allowing the patient to at least get some rest. "Engaging in behaviors other than sleep" in the bedroom allows one to be "close to the bed" in the event that the opportunity to sleep should arise and has the advantage of derailing the cognitive or physical anxiety that might occur when the patient "tries to sleep" or "worries about the next day consequences of not sleeping." From a stimulus control perspective, these practices (while highly reinforcing) set the stage for stimulus "dyscontrol"; the lowered probability that sleep related stimuli will elicit primarily sleepiness and sleep.

The therapeutic implication of this perspective is that insomnia may be treated by controlling the stimulus–response pairings so that bed, bedroom and bedtime are reassociated with the response of sleepiness and sleep. This reassociation is accomplished by creating a new conditioning history which in effect removes all but two pairings (bed and sleep, and bed and sex). Stimulus control instructions allow for the establishment of a new conditioning history by insuring that the patient does not spend protracted periods of time in the bed awake or engage in behaviors other than sleep in the bedroom. This is achieved by having the patient leave the bedroom when awake during the night and returning only when sleepy. This aspect of the treatment is based on instrumental conditioning principles. The patient engages in a voluntary behavior (get up and leave the bedroom)

and this is likely maintained by a variety of reinforcers including when the patient returns to bed and falls asleep quickly.

It is also likely that the practice of stimulus control may lead to improved sleep through classical conditioning and by the inadvertent manipulation of factors that are not behavioral. In the case of the former, the repeated pairing of bed/bedroom/bedtime with the physiologic state of sleep may allow for a counter-conditioning where sleep related stimuli elicit sleepiness and sleep due to the repeated pairing of the sleep related stimuli with the physiologic/central nervous system state of sleep. In the case of the latter, the practice of stimulus control also necessarily influences the homeostatic* and circadian† regulation of sleep.

Leaving the bedroom when awake is likely to influence the sleep homeostat. That is, when practicing stimulus control, patients are likely to lose more sleep than they would have had they stayed in bed. This sleep loss, like sleep restriction, increases sleepiness and sets the stage for strengthening of the association between the sign stimuli for sleep and sleep. Regularizing one's sleep schedule is likely to exert an influence on the patient's circadian system. That is, when practicing stimulus control there is likely to be a better alignment between the preferred sleep phase and the physiology of sleep. This alignment is likely to directly promote good sleep and probably reinforces good circadian entrainment.

SCT, while generally well tolerated, may be contraindicated for some individuals, such as those with mania, epilepsy, and parasomnias, or those who are at risk for falls. With respect to mania and epilepsy, the sleep loss that may come with this therapy may induce mania or reduce seizure threshold in at risk individuals. With respect to parasomnias, SCT related sleep loss may sufficiently deepen sleep as to increase the likelihood of partial arousal phenomenon like night terrors, sleepwalking and sleeptalking.

Sleep Restriction Therapy (SRT)

This treatment modality is also recommended for both sleep initiation and maintenance problems. Unlike stimulus control therapy, there have been relatively few evaluations in which sleep restriction is assessed as a monotherapy. As result, the American Academy of Sleep Medicine suggests that this intervention be considered "optional." While such a designation is consistent with the Sackett algorithm used by the Academy to assess what constitutes "empirical validation" (21), most behavioral sleep medicine specialists consider the intervention to be an integral part of CBT-I; 30% to 50% of the studies used to evaluate clinical efficacy of CBT-I include sleep

---

* The homeostatic regulation of sleep refers to the build up in the drive for sleep based on the prolongation of wakefulness.
† The Circadian regulation of sleep refers the neurobiologic mechanism that is thought to be the "internal clock" and responsible for pacing biological or behavioral phenomena over the course of a 24-hour day.

restriction therapy in the treatment regimens (20), and the two most recent CBT-I clinical trials (3;5) (which are the largest and most rigorous undertaken to date) also include sleep restriction therapy. Thus, while the independent effects of this intervention are not well established, it is clear that SRT is considered an essential component of CBT-I.

Sleep restriction therapy requires patients to limit the amount of time they spend in bed to an amount equal to their average total sleep time. In order to accomplish this, the clinician works with the patient to (1) establish a fixed wake time and (2) decrease sleep opportunity by limiting the subject's time in bed (TIB) to an amount that equals their average total sleep time (TST) as ascertained by baseline sleep diary measures. The standard form of this therapy recommends that the restriction be no less than 4.5 hours.

Once a target amount of time in bed is set, the patient's bedtime is delayed to later in the night so that the TIB and average TST are the same. Initially, this intervention results in mild to moderate sleep loss. This controlled form of sleep deprivation (partial sleep deprivation) usually corresponds to a decrease in sleep latency and wake after sleep onset time. Thus, during the acute phase of treatment, patients get less sleep, but they sleep in a more consolidated fashion (i.e., they fall asleep more quickly and stay asleep for longer periods of time). As sleep efficiency increases, patients are instructed to gradually increase the amount of time they spend in bed. Upward titration is accomplished in 15-minute increments; given sleep diary data that shows that for the prior week the patient's sleep was efficient (90% or more of the time spent in bed was spent asleep [TST/TIB]). See Figure 3.1 for a schematic representation of this intervention. See Appendix 1 for a detailed explanation regarding the calculation of sleep efficiency.

Three points merit further comment. First, TIB is manipulated by phase delaying the patient's sleep period (delaying bedtime). This, along with keeping a fixed wake time, results in sleep restriction. It is plausible, however, that TIB be altered by having the subject wake up at an earlier time (phase advancing wake time). This approach is not adopted because fixing "wake up time" at an earlier hour:

- Does not take advantage of the "curative" effects of delaying the sleep phase so that it corresponds to the time that is most facilitative of sleep. That is, in the effort to obtain more sleep, many patients begin to go to bed earlier and earlier. One of the effects of this strategy is to move their sleep period outside of the window of time where the biological imperative (circadian predisposition) for sleep is the strongest
- May reinforce the tendency for early morning awakenings, and
- Undermines the opportunity to pair "sleep" with "the bedtime/bedroom/bed."

Second, clinicians vary on several of the methodologic aspects of SRT. The original formulation allows patients a 15-minute increase in TIB only if

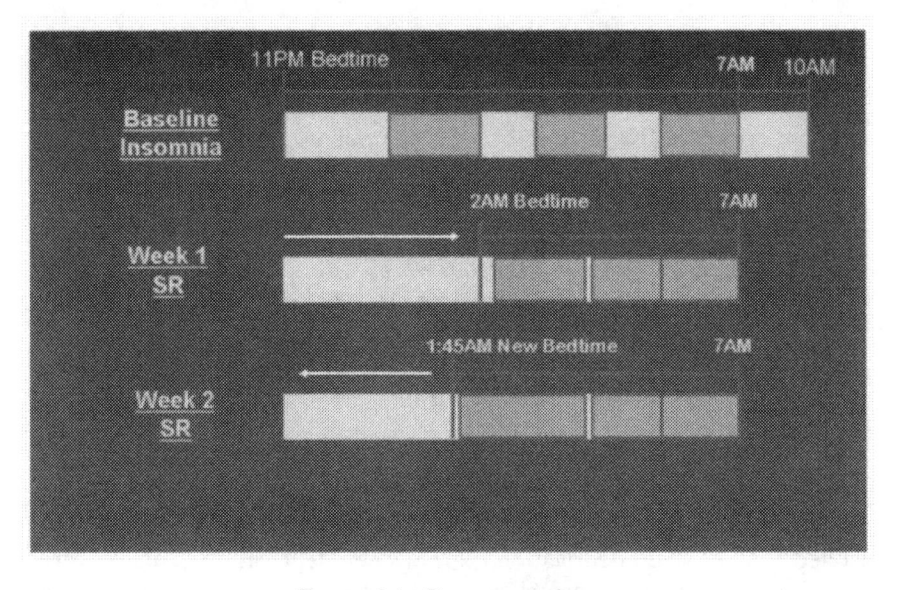

FIGURE 3.1. Sleep restriction.

their sleep is 90% sleep efficient over the course of one week. An 85% to 90% sleep efficiency results in no upward titration, and below 85% results in a 15-minute downward titration. Several variations are, however, possible. For example, the higher cutoff could be set at 85%, or the prescribed increment or decrement could be more than 15 minutes, or upward titration could be accomplished on a schedule that is shorter or longer than weekly intervals. Such variations have not been systematically researched. Therefore, for the purposes of this manual, the standard approach is adopted.

Third, it should be noted that SRT has a couple of paradoxical aspects to it. One paradox is that patients who report "not getting enough sleep" are, in essence, being told to "sleep less." The other paradox occurs over the course of treatment. With therapy, patients find that it is difficult to stay awake until the prescribed hour. This, if not paradoxical, is at least ironic for the patient that initially presents with sleep onset difficulties.

SRT is thought to be effective for two reasons. First, it prevents patients from coping with their insomnia by extending sleep opportunity. This compensatory strategy, while increasing the opportunity to get more sleep, produces a form of sleep that is shallow and fragmented. Second, the initial sleep loss that occurs with SRT is also thought to increase the homeostatic pressure for sleep, which in turn produces shorter sleep latencies, less wake after sleep onset, and higher sleep efficiency.

Finally, it should be noted that sleep restriction may also be contraindicated in patients with histories of mania, obstructive sleep aprea, seizure disorder, parasomnias or for those at risk for falls.

Sleep Hygiene Education

Sleep Hygiene Education is recommended, along with SRT and SCT, for both sleep initiation and maintenance problems. It may also have some value as a means towards increasing total sleep time. This intervention is not thought to be an effective "monotherapy" (21), but is nonetheless generally considered an integral part of CBT-I. As one might guess, Sleep hygiene is a psychoeducational intervention. Therapy most often involves providing the patient with a handout and then reviewing the items and the rationales for them. A typical set of Sleep Hygiene instructions is provided on the next page in Table 3.1.

Sleep hygiene is thought to addresses a variety of behaviors that may influence sleep quality and quantity. Its usefulness, however, may be realized when provided as part of a comprehensive approach. When combined with other treatments, the efficacy of sleep hygiene instructions may or may not be related to the absolute veracity of the various prescriptions. Instead, the value of the intervention may be in how these prescriptions (1) are tailored to the individual case, (2) allow patients to increase their knowledge about sleep, and (3) may increase compliance by enhancing the therapeutic alliance.

Second-Line Interventions (Adjunctive Treatments and Alternative-Experimental Interventions)

The therapies described below are widely not considered first-line treatments *and* are often not included in multicomponent therapy. The relegation of these treatments to the "second-line" is, in some cases, because the treatment was not found to be effective as a monotherapy and in other cases simply because there is not adequate empirical data on the intervention— as a monotherapy. The second-line treatments are summarized here so that the clinician may include these components on an as-needed basis. These interventions may be useful as adjunctive treatments that may be deployed during the second half of therapy to (1) bolster incomplete treatment responses and (2) address the predisposing and precipitating factors that are thought to still be substantially contributory.

Adjunctive/Adjuvant Therapies

Cognitive Therapy

This type of intervention is most suitable for patients who are preoccupied with the potential consequences of their insomnia or for patients who complain of unwanted intrusive ideation or worry. Several forms of cognitive therapy for insomnia have been developed. Some have a didactic focus

TABLE 3.1. Sleep Hygiene Instructions

1. **Sleep only as much as you need to feel refreshed during the following day.**
   Restricting your time in bed helps consolidate and deepen your sleep. Excessively long times in bed lead to fragmented and shallow sleep. Get up at your regular time the next day, no matter how little you slept.
2. **Get up at the same time each day, 7 days a week.**
   A regular wake time in the morning leads to regular times of sleep onset and helps to set your "biological clock."
3. **Exercise regularly.**
   Schedule exercise times so that they do not occur within 3 hours of when you intend to go to bed. Exercise makes it easier to initiate sleep and deepen sleep.
4. **Make sure your bedroom is comfortable and free from light and noise.**
   A comfortable, noise-free sleep environment will reduce the likelihood that you will wake up during the night. Noise that does not awaken you may also disturb the quality of your sleep. Carpeting, insulated curtains, and closing the door may help.
5. **Make sure that your bedroom is at a comfortable temperature during the night.**
   Excessively warm or cold sleep environments may disturb sleep.
6. **Eat regular meals and do not go to bed hungry.**
   Hunger may disturb sleep. A light snack at bedtime (especially carbohydrates) may help sleep, but avoid greasy or "heavy" foods.
7. **Avoid excessive liquids in the evening.**
   Reducing liquid intake will minimize the need for nighttime trips to the bathroom.
8. **Cut down on all caffeine products.**
   Caffeinated beverages and foods (coffee, tea, cola, chocolate) can cause difficulty falling asleep, awakenings during the night, and shallow sleep. Even caffeine early in the day can disrupt nighttime sleep.
9. **Avoid alcohol, especially in the evening.**
   Although alcohol helps tense people fall asleep more easily, it causes awakenings later in the night.
10. **Smoking may disturb sleep.**
    Nicotine is a stimulant. Try not to smoke during the night when you have trouble sleeping.
11. **Don't take your problems to bed.**
    Plan some time earlier in the evening for working on your problems or planning the next day's activities. Worrying may interfere with initiating sleep and produce shallow sleep.
12. **Do not *try* to fall asleep.**
    This only makes the problem worse. Instead, turn on the light, leave the bedroom, and do something different like reading a book. Don't engage in stimulating activity. Return to bed only when you are sleepy.
13. **Put the clock under the bed or turn it so that you can't see it.**
    Clock watching may lead to frustration, anger, and worry which interfere with sleep.
14. **Avoid naps.**
    Staying awake during the day helps you to fall asleep at night.

(24), others use paradoxical intention (25), others employ "distraction and imagery" (26), and still others use a variety of cognitive restructuring procedures (27). While the therapies differ in their approach, all are based on the observation that patients with insomnia have negative thoughts and beliefs about their condition and its consequences. Helping patients to challenge the veracity of these beliefs is thought to decrease the anxiety and arousal associated with insomnia.

Relaxation Training

This type of intervention may be most suitable for patients who character-ize their insomnia as an "inability to relax" (e.g., the patient may say: "I feel like my heart is racing when I am trying to fall asleep"), and/or for patients who present with multiple somatic complaints (e.g., deep muscle pain, headaches, gastric problems, etc.).

There are essentially four forms of relaxation therapy. The different techniques target different physiological systems. Progressive muscle relaxation is used to diminish skeletal muscle tension (28–32). Diaphrag-matic breathing is used to induce a form of respiration that is slower, deeper, and mechanically driven from the abdomen as opposed to the thorax. (It is interesting to note that this form of respiration resembles what occurs naturally at sleep onset.) Autogenic training focuses on increasing peripheral blood flow by having subjects imagine, in a systematic way, that each of their extremities feels warm. Imagery training entails the patient selecting a relaxing image or memory and evoking the image and engaging with it from a multisensory perspective.

Most practitioners select the optimal relaxation method based upon which technique is easiest for the patient to learn, and most consistent with how the patient manifests arousal. Like cognitive techniques, learning to effectively use relaxation training often requires substantial practice. Many clinicians recommend the patient rehearse the skill during the day in addition to practicing prior to sleep. When integrating into stimulus con-trol instructions, if relaxation training causes some initial "performance anxiety," it may be best to have the patient practice in a room other than the bedroom. For additional information on the various relaxation tech-niques the reader is referred to:

Overview: Lichstein, K. L. *Clinical relaxation strategies* (1988).
PMR: Bernstein, D., Borkovec, T., Hazlett-Stevens H. *Directions in Pro-gressive Relaxation Training: A Guidebook for Helping Professionals* (2000); Benson H. & Clipper M. *The Relaxation Response* (2000).
Diaphragmatic Breathing: Smith, J. C. *Advances in ABC Relaxation: Applications and inventories* (2001); Chapter: Breathing Exercises and Relaxation States.
Autogenic Training: Schultz, J. H. & Luthe, W. *Autogenic Methods* (1969).

One final cautionary note: It should be borne in mind that some patients, especially those with a history of panic disorder or performance anxiety, might experience a paradoxical response to relaxation techniques. If this occurs with one form of relaxation, it is not necessarily the case that such a reaction will occur with other forms.

Phototherapy

Phototherapy is usually accomplished using a "lightbox" which typically generates white light, or more selectively blue spectrum light at >2,000 lux.

If the patient's insomnia has a phase-delay component (i.e., the patient prefers to go to bed late and wake up late), bright light exposure in the morning for a period of 30 minutes or more may enable them to "feel sleepy" at an earlier time in the evening. In the case where the patient's insomnia has a phase-advance component (i.e., the patient prefers to go to bed early and wake up early), bright light exposure in the late evening (e.g., 8 PM–10 PM) may enable them to stay awake until a later hour.

While many may not consider phototherapy a behavioral intervention, the use of bright light is often important to integrate into the treatment regimen. This is especially true when circadian factors appear to substantially contribute to the insomnia complaint and/or when the subject is having worse than usual problems complying with the delay in bedtime that is part-and-parcel of sleep restriction therapy.

The sleep-promoting effects of bright light may occur via several mechanisms, including shifting the circadian system, enhancement of the amplitude of the circadian pacemaker, promoting wakefulness during the day, promoting alertness in the evening, or indirectly, through phototherapy's antidepressant effects (33–35).

It is generally assumed that phototherapy has no significant side effects, but this is not always the case. Severe mania has been triggered by bright light, but rarely, if ever, in patients not previously diagnosed with bipolar mood disorder. Other at risk individuals include patients with hypomania, seizure disorders, chronic headaches, eye conditions, or on medications known to cause photosensitivity. It is important to note that improper timing or duration of treatment may lead directly to an exacerbation of the illness one is seeking to treat. Accordingly, the effort to conduct this form of therapy should be informed by a good command of the extant literature (36–42).

Sleep Compression

This treatment modality is very similar to sleep restriction therapy, except that the "restriction" is done according to a graded, downward titration schedule. The restriction can be accomplished by either phase delaying bedtime or phase advancing wake time. In this way, time in bed is gradually compressed until the patient reaches the criterion level of total sleep time. Like with SRT, this treatment incrementally changes TIB over a series of weeks. Unlike SRT, the reduction is not immediate but rather occurs over a pre-specified period of time. The increment reduction is based on the average difference between TST and TIB divided by 5. Thus, over a period of five weeks, the patient is restricted to a TIB that would, under SRT, be prescribed for the first week of treatment. This form of "sleep restriction" may be ideal for patients for whom a reduced TIB is *the goal of therapy* (e.g., patients with virtually "normal" total sleep times but who have mild to moderately low sleep efficiencies). Alternatively, this approach may be

particularly ideal for patients who cannot tolerate the sudden reduction in total sleep time that occurs with SRT (28). Finally, the approach might be modified such that downward titration is discontinued prior to the five week bench mark provided that an 85% to 90% sleep efficiency is achieved. In sum, sleep compression might be thought of as a "kinder and gentler" form of sleep restriction.

Alternative-Experimental Intervention: Neurofeedback

Recently, Kayumov and colleagues (2003) (43) developed a form of neuro-feedback as a treatment for insomnia. The signal itself is based on the spectral profile of the EEG data obtained from subjects while relaxed with their eyes shut. The EEG spectral data is manipulated so that changes in the ratios of fast/slow activity are patterned to sound like music. The preliminary results from pilot studies of this technique (real versus faux feedback) suggest that patterned neurofeedback that is tailored to the individual (versus neurofeedback obtained from a subject other than the patient) produces robust changes in sleep continuity. Whether this represents a novel form of relaxation training or a form of neural conditioning or neural entrainment remains to be determined. The failure of the faux condition to produce significant prepost change, however, suggests this form of neurofeedback may indeed directly influence brain activity so as to produce improved PSG measured sleep.

Course of Treatment

The therapeutic regimen generally requires 4 to 8 weeks time with once a week face-to-face meetings with the clinical provider. Sessions range from 30 to 90 minutes depending on the stage of treatment and the degree of patient compliance. This manual describes individual treatment. There are, however, data to suggest that the group venue produces similar outcomes (44). Ultimately it may be the case that a combined approach is the most useful. That is, the first 2 to 3 sessions are undertaken on an individual basis, the middle sessions are done as group interventions, and the final session or two revert back to individual treatment. The advantage of such a regimen may be that the group setting allows for a support system for the patient and may increase compliance "by example."

Intake sessions are usually 60 to 90 minutes in duration. During this session, the clinical history is obtained and the patient is instructed in the use of sleep diaries. No intervention is provided during the first session. This time frame (usually 1–2 weeks) is used to collect the baseline sleep–wake data that will guide treatment for the balance of therapy. The primary interventions (stimulus control and sleep restriction) are deployed over the course of the next one to two 60-minute sessions. Once these treatments

are delivered, the patient enters into a phase of treatment where time in bed is upwardly titrated over the course of the next two to five visits. These follow-up sessions require about 30 minutes, unless additional interventions are being integrated into the treatment program. In the case of the present protocol, one session of Cognitive Therapy is provided at Session 5. The last one to two sessions also contain components that are devoted to maintaining wellness and what to do when relapses occur.

Which Patients are Appropriate for CBT-I

Therapists should never assume all patients referred to them for insomnia treatment have been accurately diagnosed. It is entirely possible that the insomnia is part of an unstable and/or undiagnosed intrinsic sleep disorder (other than insomnia), medical illness, or psychiatric illness. Thus, it is important that the clinician first determine whether the patient is appropriate for treatment. The easiest determination is in the instances where the patient presents with primary, or psychophysiologic, insomnia. Limiting treatment to this population, however, may be too restrictive. While a matter of some debate, most would agree (regardless of diagnosis) that the appropriate patients for CBT-I are people who present with:

- difficulty falling or staying asleep
- a report of one or more of the following
  —regularly extend their sleep opportunity to compensate for sleep loss and/or
  —stay in bed for protracted periods of time while awake and/or
  —engage in behaviors other than sleep and sex in the bedroom
- evidence of conditioned arousal, e.g., the report of being suddenly awake when getting into bed and/or sleeping better when away from home (optional)
- evidence of poor sleep hygiene [the engagement of behaviors that reduce sleep propensity, e.g., use of alcohol as a hypnotic, stimulant use at night (optional)].

The controversy is that some would suggest that when the insomnia is thought to be secondary to a medical or psychiatric condition, then treatment for the primary condition is the sole indication; the concept being that once the primary condition is treated, the secondary insomnia will resolve. This implies that CBT-I is not indicated in such cases. It has recently been suggested, however, that the distinction between primary and secondary insomnia is not easily made (45–47) and there is a growing body of literature which suggests that so-called "secondary insomnia" may be equally responsive to CBT-I (48–54).

One way of understanding why the distinction between primary and secondary insomnia may be less important is to consider the issue by taking

into account the Behavioral Model of Insomnia as put forward by Spielman and colleagues (17). For a diagram of the Behavioral Model, see Figure 2.1. As indicated previously, this model suggests that acute medical and/or psychiatric illness may precipitate an acute bout of insomnia, but when the parent disorder is diagnosed, treated, and/or stable, the persistent (or residual) insomnia is likely to be more like primary insomnia than the insomnia that accompanied the acute illness. That is, the residual insomnia and/or chronic insomnia is likely to be maintained by factors other than those that precipitated the acute episode. Thus, if there is evidence that the insomnia is maintained by behavioral factors and/or there is evidence of conditioned arousal and/or poor sleep hygiene, the patient is likely to be a good candidate for CBT-I, so long as the "primary" disorder is not neglected. How these factors are assayed will be addressed in the section devoted to Session 1 (The Intake Interview).

Which Clinicians Are Appropriate for CBT-I

Traditionally, CBT-I and/or CBT for other sleep disorders have been developed, and provided, by psychologists. In addition, CBT-I providers usually have clinical degrees and speciality training in sleep medicine, behavioral medicine, and/or cognitive behavioral therapy. Training in each of these areas is critical. A thorough grounding in sleep medicine allows the clinician to be attuned to the presence of occult sleep and medical disorders. An expertise in behavioral medicine and cognitive behavioral therapy allows the clinician (in general) a broad understanding of principles and practice of behavioral treatments and (in specific) the ability to conduct behavioral assessments (e.g., contingency analyses). In addition, the individual with behavioral medicine and/or cognitive behavioral therapy expertise is likely to be well versed in psychological assessment and the diagnosis and treatment of psychiatric disorders, and is likely to subscribe to a philosophy that emphasizes the use of empirically validated treatment.

As the field matures, it is likely that physicians and psychologists from related fields will wish to integrate behavioral sleep medicine interventions into their practices or to develop a specialized expertise in this area. It is hoped that the information provided in this manual will serve as a useful entrée. It is expected that expertise in the area can only be achieved with dedicated training (e.g., pre- or postdoctoral fellowships) or at minimum apprenticeship and/or peer supervision. It is also likely that individuals with non-doctoral clinical degrees may want to incorporate CBT-I into their work. Again the expectation is that the information provided in this manual will serve as a useful entrée and that good practice dictates the need for further supervision.

Finally, it should be noted that as of June 2003, there is a board dedicated to credentialing specialists in behavioral sleep medicine. Currently, this cer-

tification is offered by the American Academy of Sleep Medicine (AASM) and is open to PhD- and MD-level licensed clinicians. In the future, it may be the case that masters-level licensed clinicians may be eligible for a related certification. While it may be some time before such credentials are required for provision of treatment and reimbursement for services, it is important to be aware that these qualifications may soon be required to be deemed an expert. This is particularly important for younger clinicians who are just beginning training in this area. For further information on Behavioral Sleep Medicine Certification, please visit the American Academy of Sleep Medicine's Web site at www.aasmnet.org. Specific information about exam eligibility and the BSM exam itself can be found at www.aasmnet.org/behavioralexam.asp.

The Clinical Relationship

There is no question that therapeutic style varies radically from therapist to therapist. What works for one may not work well for another. This said, there is a set of characteristics that is thought to make one a "good clinician." In general, this set includes good listening skills, a strong sense of empathy, respect for patient's autonomy, good persuasion skills, and perhaps a sense of humor. Specifically, the clinician needs to adopt at least two personas. On the one hand, the clinician needs to demonstrate his or her expertise in order to build patient confidence in the treatment regimen. This is particularly important in the opening phase of treatment, when the didactic element of therapy is focal (Sessions 1–4). On the other hand, the clinician needs to adopt a less directive role, particularly in the latter half of therapy. During this phase of treatment, the patient is well served by having the clinician characterize their part to play as less like a physician or psychologist, and more like a physical therapist (trainer and/or coach). Setting it up so that the patient sees both aspects of the clinician's role can be difficult, but it has the desirable outcome of making it clear to the patient who carries the responsibility for positive clinical gains in the latter half of therapy.

Another ingredient that is required for a strong therapeutic alliance is that the therapist clearly relay to the patient the likely outcomes of therapy, what is required to achieve these results, and in what time frame the patient can reasonably expect positive gains. It is important that this information not be "sugar coated." If the patient expects that therapy will be easy and without sacrifice, he is likely to be surprised and/or overwhelmed and more likely to be nonadherent or to quit therapy. It is essential that the patient understand that he will get worse before he gets better. If the patient is prepared for this experience, he is more likely to "stay with the program" and endure the initial phase of therapy. The therapeutic alliance will also be enhanced by making sure that the patient understands the rationale behind

the procedures he is to carry out. Some patients may be motivated by doing "what the doctor told them to do", but in most cases patients tend to be more adherent when they know why they are doing what they are doing.

The Clinic Environment

What is the optimal location for a behavioral sleep medicine clinic? This question is not easily answered. In many ways the ideal setting is a sleep disorders center. This allows an interdisciplinary approach to diagnosis and treatment and may be consistent with the patient's expectation about what the disorder is and where it should be treated. Clinics located in other venues may still greatly benefit by a formal affiliation with a sleep disorders center, as this will allow the clinician access to other sleep specialists (pulmonologists, neurologists, otolaryngologists, etc.) and enhance the credibility of the free-standing clinic. The association with the speciality center will, in turn, enhance the patient's view that the clinician is a sleep expert and may promote compliance with CBT-I. Clinics not affiliated with sleep disorder centers may do well to consider how else they might highlight their credentials and allay patient concerns regarding whether they will have access to knowledgeable specialists. One concrete way of addressing this is to make sure that one's brochures document the speciality nature of the clinic and the credentials of its staff. For an example of a clinic brochure, see Appendix 2.

The Clinician's Office

While most practitioners familiar with CBT know that the office environment requires certain "trade items," it is worth noting for the novitiate that some stock equipment is necessary. Treatment will require a table that is separate from the clinician's desk, a dry erase board, and possibly a reclining chair for relaxation training. The table allows a common space where the patient and clinician can collaborate. A third chair for the table may be useful when a spouse or significant other is invited to attend. The dry erase board provides the clinician the space needed to represent their points visually (e.g., portraying the Spielman Model of Insomnia, depicting sleep architecture with a hypnogram, etc.).

Clinic Chart

In general, regardless of the type of practice, the clinic chart serves two purposes: (1) to document the patient's clinical history (his past and current diagnoses) and codify the treatment plan, and (2) to provide the requisite

documentation for third party reimbursement, legal issues, and so on. For the purpose of CBT for insomnia, it can be argued that the clinic chart has a third, and more important, function. It serves as the data source for the conduct of therapy (graphs to illustrate response to treatment), program evaluation, and clinical case series research. With respect to this first point, it should be emphasized that the graphs depicting the patient's progress over time has substantial clinical utility, for both the clinician and the patient. For the clinician, the graphs (which depict weekly averages for each of the sleep diary-based measures of sleep continuity [sleep latency, wake after sleep onset, total sleep time, and sleep efficiency]) allow for an "at a glance" view of whether treatment is on target. Such information allows therapy to be "evidenced based" and provides a means towards this end that is less dependent on the content of the progress notes. For the patient, the graphs can serve as good intermediate reinforcement (evidence of forward progress). For examples of treatment graphs that illustrate a typical course of therapy, see Appendix 3.

Clinical Assessment

As with most clinical practices, CBT-I has essentially two phases: an assessment phase and a treatment phase. As with most cognitive behavioral practices, the initial assessment process has both retrospective and prospective components. The retrospective component entails the administration of questionnaires and the intake interview. The prospective component requires that patients use diaries to record their symptoms on a daily basis for one to two weeks. More information will be provided about the clinical interview in the session-by-session section that follows.

Retrospective Measures

There are, of course, an endless number of questionnaires that one could administer to gather relevant information. For clinical practice purposes one must be careful to make good use of patient contact time and not burden the patient, yet get a comprehensive profile. While the standard battery of instruments used varies from clinic to clinic, there are a handful of questionnaires that are generally administered. These "tap," at minimum, personal and family information, health and mood status, and sleep disturbance profile. Table 3.2 provides a list of instruments that allow for a reasonable retrospective assessment of the patient. The combination of these instruments allows the clinician to not only create a good clinical profile of the patient, but provides the evidence needed to decide if the patient should be referred because of undiagnosed or unstable medical or psychiatric illness. Retrospective questionnaires also provide the clinician with the patient's global attributions regarding his or her sleep and health status. Appendix 4 contains examples of the questionnaires that are typically

TABLE 3.2. Useful Questionnaires for Intake Evaluation

Name of instrument	Measure of general information	References
General information questionnaire	***	
Medical history survey	***	
Medical symptoms check list	***	
Check list of sleep disorders symptoms	***	
Psychiatric instruments		
The Beck Depression Inventory (BDI)	Global depression severity	Ambrosini et al., 1991 (84) Bumberry et al., 1978 (85) Robinson et al., 1996 (86) Schotte et al., 1997 (87)
Beck Anxiety Inventory (Alternative STAI)	Global anxiety severity.	de Beurs et al., 1997 (88) Osman et al., 1997 (89)
General health and pain information		
SF-36 Health Survey	Health profile measuring quality of life. Factor/Subscale Scores for: 1. physical functioning 2. social functioning 3. role limitations due to physical problems 4. role limitations due to emotional problems 5. mental health 6. energy/vitality 7. pain 8. general health perception	Ware et al., 1992 (90) McHorney et al., 1994 (91) Brazier et al., 1992 (92)
The Multidimensional Pain Inventory (MPI)	Comprehensive assessment of subjective pain experience. Factor/Subscale Scores for: 1. pain severity 2. interference 3. life control 4. affective distress 5. social support 6. general activity level	Kerns et al.,1985 (93) Turk & Rudy, 1988 (94)
Sleep and fatigue instruments		
The Pittsburgh Sleep Quality Index (PSQI)	Global sleep disturbance severity Factor/ Subscale Scores for: 1. subjective sleep quality 2. sleep latency 3. sleep duration 4. habitual sleep efficiency 5. sleep disturbances 6. use of sleep medication 7. daytime dysfunction	Buysse et al., 1989 (95)
The Insomnia Severity Index	Simple global measure of illness severity	Morin et al. 2001 (96)
Sleep Environment Checklist		
Epworth Sleepiness Scale (ESS)	Measure of daytime sleepiness.	Johns, 1994 (97)
Multidimensional Fatigue Inventory (MFI)	Global assessment of fatigue.	Smets et al., 1995 (98)

"home grown" (i.e. created by the clinic as needed [e.g., Medical History Checklist (4a), Symptom Checklist (4b), Sleep Disorders Symptom Checklist (4c), a Sleep Environment Checklist (4d) and Motivation for Change Index (4e)]).

Prospective Measures

The primary tool for prospective assessment is the sleep diary. It allows the clinician to (1) evaluate the severity of the insomnia on a day-to-day basis, (2) identify the behaviors that maintain the insomnia, (3) determine to what extent circadian dysrhythmia is present, and (4) gather the data needed to measure and guide treatment.

Assessment with sleep diaries requires that patients keep a daily log for a 1 to 2 week time interval so that the behaviors of interest can be sampled across time. Like retrospective measures of sleep continuity (e.g., the Pittsburgh Sleep Quality Index [PSQI] or the Insomnia Severity Index [ISI]), sleep diaries also require subjects to make estimates regarding such things as how long it takes them to fall asleep, how much time is spent awake during the night, etc. All of the traditional sleep continuity variables may be obtained with sleep diaries including sleep latency (SL), frequency of nocturnal awakenings (FNA), wake after sleep onset time (WASO), and total sleep time (TST). In addition, the sampled data may be used to track three additional parameters and to derive one additional measure.

The derived measure is referred to as sleep efficiency (SE%). This variable represents *total sleep time* as a percentage of *time in bed* (TST/TIB]*100) and allows, with a single measure, the clinician the ability to assess (1) the extent to which sleep opportunity and sleep ability are mismatched and (2) the effects of treatment. Please note that this measure may be obtained using retrospective instruments but is almost always calculated when sleep diary data are available.

The tracking variables include the prescribed "time to bed" (PTIB) and "time out of bed" (PTOB) and the "amount of time spent out of bed during the night" (i.e., during the intended sleep period (TOB)). These measures may be used to assess patient compliance (see Session 2).

Currently, there are no "industry standard" sleep-wake diaries. Two are included in the appendices as examples. One is a single page per week instrument and the other is a single page per day instrument (see Appendix 5 and 6). While both are used to record daily information for a seven-day time frame, the two formats have different advantages and disadvantages. A single page per week instrument has the advantage of being concise, compact and easy for both the patient and the clinician to use. The ease of use may also enhance compliance with the effort to obtain prospective data. The disadvantage is that the patient may be more likely to use previous entries as a cue or guide for completing new entries. For

example, the patient may see that she/he has been reporting 5-minute sleep latencies for the last few days and adjust her/his new estimate relative to these data. A single-page per day instrument has the advantage of providing more space for additional measures and is likely to be less intimidating given the single page format is more like a traditional diary. The disadvantage of this format is that the "bulk pack" of seven diaries per week may appear "work intensive" to the patient and is more difficult to use for the in-session review.

The primary difference between the retrospective and prospective measurement of sleep continuity is that the estimate obtained from the nightly sleep diary applies to only one time point (last night) and therefore does not require the patient to understand the concept of an average or encourage him to use heuristics to form and relay impressions regarding her/his sleep quantity and quality.

The primary value of obtaining nightly estimates via the use of sleep diaries is that it allows the clinician/investigator (1) to collect a reasonable sample on which he/she can calculate measures of central tendency and night-to-night variability and (2) to conduct contingency analyses. With respect to this latter point, behavioral sleep medicine specialists often sample a standard repertoire of behaviors so that they can determine whether certain traditional factors are related to the incidence and severity of insomnia symptoms. For example, does the patient nap? Does sleep latency reliably get longer on the days that the patient naps? A covariation between these measures would suggest to the therapist that the napping behavior needs to be modified or eliminated. Because many of the behavioral contingencies vis-à-vis insomnia have been well delineated (e.g., the maladaptive behaviors of extending sleep opportunity, napping, caffeine use, the use of alcohol as a sedative, etc.), these are sometimes not included on, or measured with, sleep diaries. Prospective measurement, nonetheless, allows for the engagement of broad-based contingency analysis when the need arises.

It should be noted that with the advent of the internet, PDAs, and hand held PCs, paper versions of diaries are likely to become a thing of the past. There are a plethora of advantages to the newer technologies including:

- The therapist can track via date and time stamps when the diary entries are made.
- Patients can be prompted to complete the instrument in between sessions.
- No secondary data entry is required.
- Data can be easily manipulated and displayed.
- Performance measures (e.g., reaction time tests) may be integrated into the assessment.

The Role of Polysomography

The measurement of sleep by polysomnography (PSG) allows for objective measurement, excellent temporal (moment-by-moment) resolution, direct and quantitative measures of brain and somatic activity during sleep, and the ability to resolve substates (i.e., sleep architecture) that are not apparent with other measures. Coupled with other electrophysiological measures (e.g., electrocardiograms, nasal/oral air flow, etc.) this methodology paved the way for the first observations about the medical disorders that occur during sleep (e.g., obstructive sleep apnea, periodic leg movements of sleep, etc.). Accordingly, the PSG mode of assessment is the "gold standard" for sleep research and neurologic and pulmonary sleep medicine. While polysomnography is not considered integral to the direct practice of Behavioral Sleep Medicine, knowledge about the measure is required so that behavioral specialists can make good use of these data when available and better interface with other sleep medicine specialists.

The primary advantage of PSG over self-report and actigraphy (see below) is that this measure reveals that sleep is not a unitary state. That is, sleep is not something that one is either "in" or "not in." Interestingly, even introspection would lead us to this conclusion. Certainly, it feels true that there is "shallow" and "deep" sleep and "dream" and "not-dream" sleep. This alone suggests that there are 2 to 4 stages or states of sleep. With the advent of polysomnography, it was found that such impressions are indeed rooted in something that can be objectively measured.

PSG, as it is used to define states of consciousness, is comprised of three measures: electroencephalography (EEG), electromyography (EMG), and electroocculography (EOG). Each of these measures, while based on different source potentials, capitalizes on naturally occurring electrical currents that are radiated from the scalp, muscles, and eyes. These currents can be represented continuously and plotted over time. Such graphs provide a moment-by-moment view of brain, motor, and eye movement activity. The combination of these plots allows for the detection and categorization of no less than five stages of sleep (Stages 1–4 & REM sleep).

At this time, it is not believed that patients with primary insomnia exhibit clinically relevant sleep architectural abnormalities (abnormal proportions of one or more of the stages of sleep), neither do they exhibit the kind of cardiopulmonary abnormalities that are observed with PSG and account for other types of intrinsic sleep disorders (e.g., obstructive sleep apnea, period limb movements of sleep). Thus, PSG is not currently indicated for the assessment of primary, or secondary, insomnia. If, however, the patient is not responsive to CBT-I or pharmacologic treatment, PSG follow-up is usually warranted and the procedure may reveal occult disorders (intrinsic sleep disorders for which the typical signs and symptoms are not present on clinical interview). For example, if one allows for the complaint of non-restorative sleep to be synonymous with (or an example of) insomnia, PSG

may reveal an underlying pathology known as "Alpha-Delta" sleep (also referred to as simply alpha sleep).

The Role of Actigraphy

Actigraphy allows for the objective assessment of sleep continuity parameters. The methodology uses motion detection and activity counts to assess whether the patient is awake or asleep. The actigraphic device itself resembles a wristwatch and the output data can be summarized graphically as activity counts over time or quantitatively. The device and an example of an output report are pictured in Figure 3.2.

While the algorhithms that are applied to make these determinations are quite sophisticated, the central idea is that "when the subject is moving, they are awake" and "when subject is immobile, they are asleep." The device produces minute-by-minute data that ultimately allows for the calculation of the usual compliment of sleep continuity variables. The primary strengths of this prospective measurement strategy are that it (1) allows for an assessment of sleep continuity that is free from either self report or observer bias, (2) requires minimal subject compliance, (3) has excellent temporal resolution (allows for the detection of periods of wakefulness as brief as 30 seconds in duration), (4) allows for the continuous assessment for periods of up to 60 days, (5) when combined with sleep diary data may allow for the detection of "sleep state misperception" (a condition where subjects appear by objective measures to be asleep but do not perceive themselves to be asleep), (6) may cause the patient to more veridically report their sleep continuity in the sleep diaries, and (7) may provide a measure of compliance with the prescribed aspects of treatment (prohibition against napping, and schedule bedtime and awake time).

To date, actigraphy is not a standard procedure for the initial assessment, the measure of treatment compliance, or the evaluation of treatment change. This is unfortunate as this measurement strategy may richly inform each of these areas. In the assessment phase, actigraphy may be used to identify circadian rhythm abnormalities (e.g., phase shifts, free running rhythms, etc.) and subjects who have a larger degree of sleep state misperception (now referred to as paradoxical insomnia). While this latter application has yet to be validated (i.e., does the combination of sleep diaries and actigraphy yield a comparable measure of sleep state misperception as it is derived with sleep diaries and polysomnography?), our sense is that the combination of sleep diaries and actigraphy may be used to alert the clinician to the fact that sleep state misperception is a significant component of the patient's clinical profile. If this is the case, one may expect, in the absence of empirical data on this subject, that such a patient may be less responsive to standard treatment.

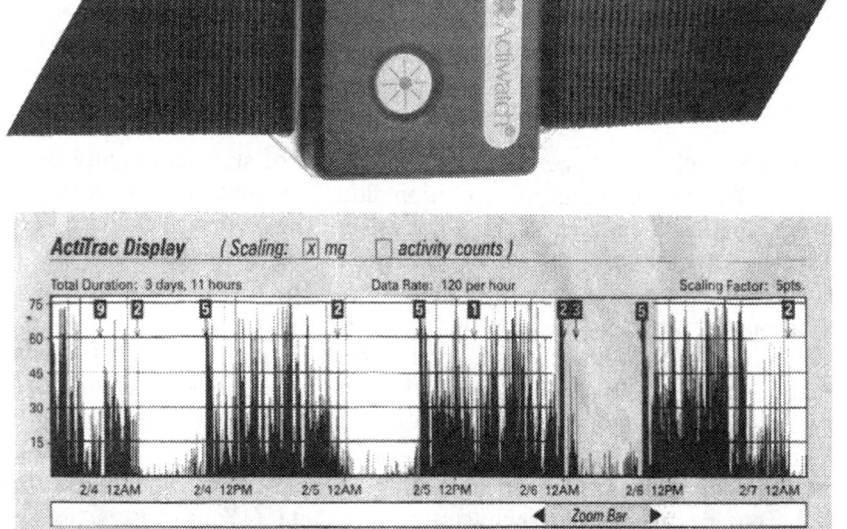

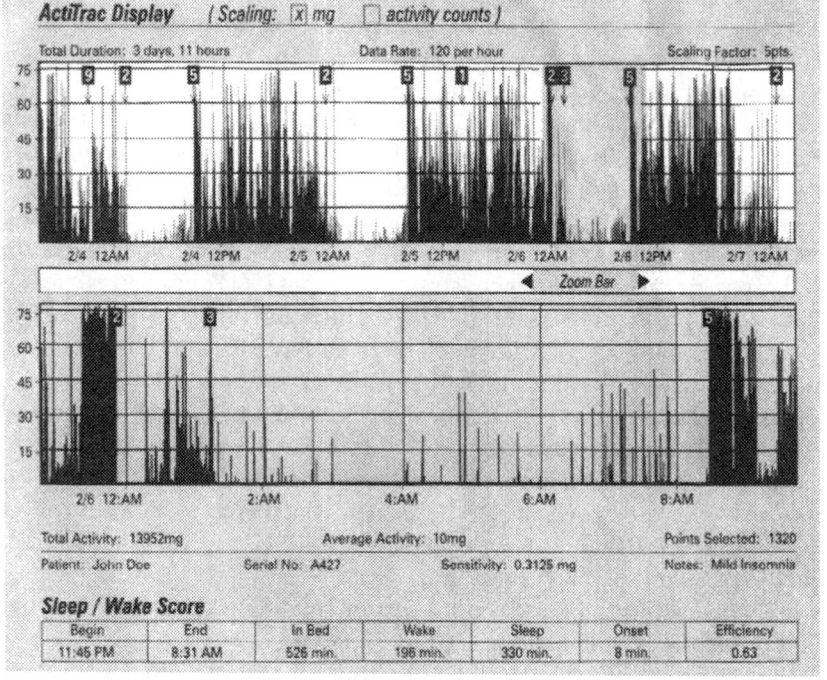

Figure 3.2. Actigraphs (Photographs provided by Mini Mitter Co., Mini Mitter Co., Inc., 20300 Empire Avenue, Building B-3, Bend, Oregon 97701).

In the treatment phase, actigraphy may be used to objectively assess sleep continuity gains and to determine if the patient is being adherent. With respect to the latter, actigraphy may be used to document that the patient has complied with the prescribed phase delay in bedtime, with the prohibition against napping during the day, and with prescriptions to get out of bed (1) during the night when awake (stimulus control) and (2) at the appointed hour in the morning.

For the purposes of this treatment manual, we'll assume that such devices are available only on a limited basis and thus used primarily for the assess-

ment of sleep state misperception and adherence (in the cases which warrant such evaluations) and with patients who are unable to keep a sleep diary.

First Patient Contact

How patients come to seek, or be referred to, behavioral sleep medicine services is quite variable. Some patients may self-refer, some may be triaged from clinical research trials, some may be referred from local sleep disorders centers, while still others may be referred by their medical provider. "First contact" is, more often than not, with secretarial staff or answering services. Some clinics may elect to undertake superficial screens at this level to insure that the patient is an appropriate candidate for treatment. Alternatively, "first contact" can be limited to obtaining an address and sending a brochure to the prospective patient. The advantage of the latter strategy is that, for the patients that have a medical bias regarding their diagnosis and treatment, this will provide an opportunity for them to acclimate to the idea of a "behavioral service."

Some services may make use of the internet to provide or obtain preliminary information. The advantage to such a format is that some or all of the retrospective questionnaires may be obtained in this manner. In most cases, however, the primary value of such a "portal" is for research protocols that need to screen patients as opposed to clinical services that might provide better service via face-to-face contacts. While currently configured as a research instrument, an example of a Web-based survey instrument may be found at www.sleeplessinrochester.com.

4
CBT-I Session by Session

Session One: Intake Evaluation (60 to 120 Minutes)

Tasks

Introduce Yourself to the Patient
Complete Intake Questionnaires
Conduct Clinical Interview
Determine If Patient Is a Candidate for CBT-I
Determine Other Treatment Options
Present an Overview of Treatment Options
Orient Patient to the Sleep Diary (and actigraph)
Field Patient Questions and Address Resistances
Setting the Weekly Agenda

Primary Goals of This Session

1. Identify whether the patient has an unstable or undiagnosed medical or psychiatric disorder.
2. Determine if the insomnia is precipitated and/or maintained by substance use/abuse or by the iatrogenic effects of concomitant medications.
3. Establish that the CBT-I is indicated.
4. Describe the approach, its efficacy, and provide an overview of the program.
5. Decide with the patient if "this is a good time" to invest the time and effort needed for Tx.
6. For patients using OTC or prescription sleep medications, determine whether they are willing to discontinue the use of these agents and explain the possible strategies.
7. Orient the patient to the process of keeping a sleep diary. If actigraphs are being used, orient the patient to the use of the actigraph. Explain why both measures are used.

8. Explain why baseline data is needed. Encourage the patient to not alter their schedule or habits in any way.

Introduce Yourself to the Patient

Foolish as it may seem to put this on the "to-do" list, the first contact is a critical series of moments during which the patient is likely to be deciding "whether you're the right person for the job." While we can only speculate what factors go into this judgment, our sense is that the clinician should approach the patient in a friendly, warm, and maybe even casual manner, but take charge immediately by establishing his/her credentials and the agenda for the session. For example:

Dialogue #2: Therapist Introduces Self to Patient

Therapist: Hello Mr. Jones, My name is Dr. Smith. I am the senior clinician with the service. and I'll be working with you today to evaluate your sleep problem. Over the course of today's appointment we're going to begin the process of figuring out if your insomnia is what it seems, and whether our service is appropriate for you. To do this, we'll need you to complete some questionnaires. . . . We'll review these together and then figure out the next steps.

In most cases, the next step requires that we meet for another session, and that between now and then both you and I have some additional information to gather. My part will require that I check in with your primary care clinician (and/or your psychiatrist) to make sure that nothing has been missed . . . and I'll need to spend some time formulating what will be the best treatment plan for you. Your part will require that you help us characterize your insomnia more comprehensively using a sleep diary (and an actigraph). At the end of the session we'll talk more about this—and why such information is needed.

Okay. Lets get you started working on these background surveys. If you have any questions, please feel free to ask. Also, please know in advance, that some of the questionnaires may pose some fairly personal questions. It is important that you answer these as honestly as you can. As you complete each survey, please pass it to me so I can look over your answers.

Complete Intake Questionnaires and Administer an Insomnia Severity Index

In the clinical setting, one may elect to have the patient complete the battery of questionnaires at home or in the waiting room. If the clinic staff

is providing the materials to the patient in the waiting room, whoever provides the packet should be sure to explain the purpose of the "bulk pack" of questionnaires. In the case where the questionnaires are completed at home (on paper or by PC), a cover letter should be used to provide the above information.

The up side of "home administration" is that the patient can accomplish the task in the comfort of her/his own home, do the paper work at her/his own speed, and when she comes to clinic, the information is already collected. The down side of the "home administration" is the patient is unable to ask questions about the materials and/or she/he may be less attentive to the task, given the distractions of being at home. For the purposes of this manual, it will be assumed that the paperwork is administered in clinic and with the treating clinician present.

Conduct Clinical Interview and Determine If Patient Is a Candidate for CBT-I

As indicated above, in our program the clinician reviews the material as the patient is completing each instrument. This allows the clinician to flag items that bear on the central issues for the interview. In a very real sense, the central issues are a matter of determining whether the patient meets the inclusion and exclusion criteria for treatment. When conducting clinical trials, failing to meet an inclusion criteria or meeting an exclusion criteria will necessitate that the patient be referred elsewhere. In clinical practice, the determination to treat or not treat is more complex.

The structure for the following sections (the indications and contraindications for CBT-I) adopts a practical but non-traditional approach. Instead of making the determination regarding whether treatment is indicated on the basis of diagnosis, we provide a framework or an algorithm for this determination (see Figure 4.1). The algorrithm determines (1) whether the patient exhibits the factors that are targeted by CBT-I and (2) whether CBT-I is contraindicated because of the presence of confounding issues.

The Indications for CBT-I

The simplest approach is to first establish that CBT-I *may be* indicated. This can be done by establishing the following bench marks:

- *Does the patient have substantial sleep continuity problems (Disorders of Initiation and Maintenance [DIMS])?*
  Does it take the patient 30 or more minutes to fall asleep?
  Does the patient spend 30 or more minutes awake over the course of the night?
  Do these difficulties occur regularly throughout the week (3 or more nights per week)?

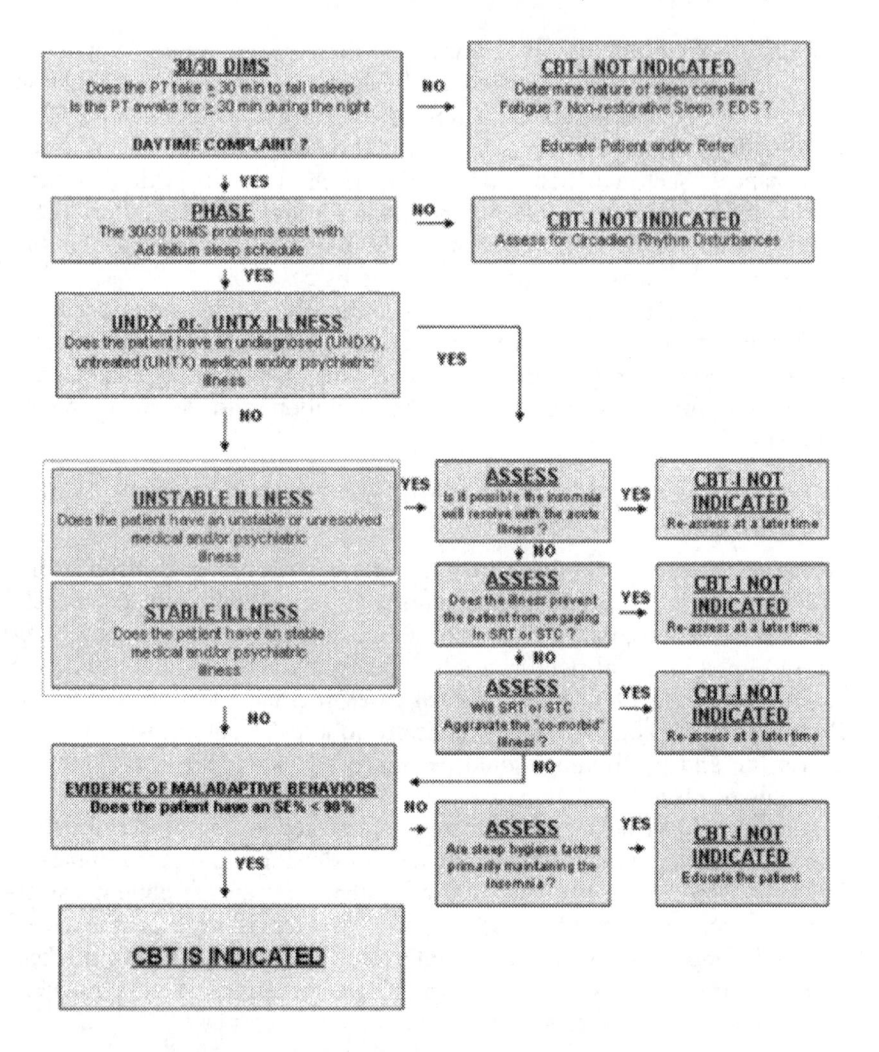

FIGURE 4.1. Assessment Algorithm: Is CBT-I Indicated?

How precisely one applies the "30-minute rule" depends largely on the context for treatment. Research protocols may follow a rigid application of the rule. In practice there a variety of considerations where the patient may not meet the severity criteria and yet CBT-I may still be indicated.

Values of less than 30 minutes and/or less than 3 days per week (as measured by, e.g., the clinic's "home-grown" sleep survey instrument or the PSQI and/or the ISI [See Table 3.2]) may suggest that the patient's primary concerns are related to the problem of nonrestorative or fragmented sleep. Such a profile often suggests that an intrinsic sleep disorder (other than insomnia) may be present and a referral for polysomnography may be war-

ranted. This need not, however, always be the case. For example, it is not uncommon to have a patient who has already undergone a PSG evaluation and who has been found to have nonrestorative and/or fragmented sleep which is not ascribable to sleep disordered breathing or other organic sleep disturbances. Such a patient may benefit from sleep restriction therapy despite the fact that she/he has not met the traditional severity criteria. This example underscores the need for multidisciplinary evaluation and the importance of evaluating patients on a case by case basis.

Irrespective of severity criteria, sleep continuity problems that occur *on fewer than 3 days per week* may or may not require CBT-I, but certainly warrant a contingency analyses to determine if situational factors are responsible for the occurrence of the initiation and or maintenance problems.

- *Does the patient report that her/his daytime function is compromised because of their insomnia?*

Assessing whether or not there are impairments can often be difficult. Many patients with long-term insomnia have learned to cope with the consequences of the insomnia. This may be so much the case that the patient, in the face of substantial sleep continuity problems, actually denies that she suffers daytime consequences. In such cases, it is useful to probe further. Rather than ask about deficits, it is useful to ask the patient what aspects of her life and functioning would be improved if her sleep problem was suddenly resolved.

Daytime impairment and/or distress is assessed so that one can determine whether the patient is naturally a short sleeper and that the apparent insomnia is occurring because of a mismatch between the patient's sleep schedule and sleep need. Another possibility regarding the absence of daytime complaints, is that the patient's sleep need is reduced for medical and/or psychiatric reasons. As with the above scenario, further assessment and diagnostic work is required.

- *Is there evidence that the insomnia is maintained by behavioral factors?*

One can identify the maintaining or behavioral factors (compensatory strategies) by single item questions on surveys or by direct questions on interview. A relatively comprehensive list of maintaining factors and compensatory strategies are contained in Table 4.1.

Perhaps the most common of the compensatory strategies, and those primarily targeted by CBT-I, are as follows. "As the insomnia got worse, did you deal with your fatigue (or catch up for lost sleep) by

- going to bed earlier?
- sleeping in?
- regularly napping during the day?"

Each of these behaviors represent the effort to extend sleep opportunity in the face of sleep loss. This strategy, as valid as it may seem, results in the

TABLE 4.1. Perpetuating Factors of Insomnia

Compensatory strategy	Effect on sleep
Extending sleep opportunity	
Go to bed early	Deprimes "sleep homeostat" leading to insomnia and shallow sleep. Possible circadian dysregulation
Sleep in (wake up later)	Deprimes "sleep homeostat" Possible circadian dysregulation
Napping	Deprimes "sleep homeostat."
Counter fatigue measures	
Increased use of stimulants and/or inappropriately-timed use of stimulants	Increases sleep interfering states of arousal.
Avoid or decrease physical activity	May de-prime "sleep homeostat." Can lead to conditioned arousal if increased time spent resting in bed or in bedroom.
Rituals and strategies	
Increase in nonsleep behaviors in the bedroom to "kill time"	Promotes a lack of stimulus control.
Sleep somewhere other than the bedroom	Promotes a lack of stimulus control.
Engage in "rituals" which are thought to promote sleep (use of special herbs, teas, etc.)	Promotes a dependence on the behaviors and anticipatory anxiety when not available.
Avoidance of behaviors thought to inhibit sleep (e.g., sex, going outdoors near bedtime, etc.)	Promotes anticipatory anxiety when behaviors occur.
Self-medication strategies (sedation)	
Increased alcohol intake, qhs	REM suppression and rebound sleep fragmentation, early morning awakenings. Decreased sleep-related self-efficacy.
Marijuana use	Effects on sleep are poorly understood; discontinuation/withdrawal may exacerbate the insomnia. Decreased sleep-related self-efficacy.
Overuse of OCT sedatives (antihistamines)	Increase psychological dependence on medication to sleep. Decreased sleep-related self-efficacy, morning hangover.
Melatonin used as a hypnotic	May induce circadian phase shifts, which may promote the insomnia. Increase psychological dependence on substance to sleep. Decreased sleep-related self-efficacy. May have a within or across night withdraw and rebound insomnia. Lack of FDA regulation.

dysregulation of the "sleep homeostat." That is, when one "sleeps in" or goes to bed early, this may compensate for prior sleep loss, but has the unintended effect of decreasing the amount of time spent awake. This reduction in time spent awake means that the individual is more sleep satiated on the next occasion on which she/he seeks to sleep. This reduction in "sleep pres-

sure" is referred to as depriming the sleep homeostat. The consequence is an increased probability that the patient will have difficulty initiating and/or maintaining sleep on the occasion following the days where the patient compensated for her sleep loss. In the long run, this form of sleep dysregulation is thought to, in and of itself, perpetuate insomnia. As indicated above, this "effect" may be quantified using a single measure which depicts the tendency to increase sleep opportunity in the face of sleep loss. This variable is referred to as sleep efficiency (SE%). Sleep efficiencies of <85% suggests that there is a behaviorally maintained mismatch between sleep opportunity and sleep "ability." Sleep efficiencies of 90% or greater may suggest, as above, that the patient's primary complaints are not so much related to insomnia as they are to psychosocial factors, the problem of nonrestorative sleep, insufficient sleep syndrome, or other sleep, medical, or psychiatric disorders. Please note that it is possible that some patients may have low sleep efficiency without having engaged in extending sleep opportunity. While this tends to be characteristic of acute insomnia or insomnias secondary to medical or psychiatric conditions or insomnias related to other intrinsic sleep disorders, these "nonprimary" insomnias may also benefit from CBT-I.

Of the above considerations, one factor or clinical consideration is notably absent. The factor not listed pertains to illness chronicity. While important for the full characterization of the clinical disorder (especially if one is attempting to define insomnia in a way that approximates a Research Diagnostic Criteria based definition), it is not essential for the determination of whether CBT-I is indicated. This said, it may be relevant for whether CBT-I is contraindicated (see below). In many ways, "how long one has had insomnia" is a proxy variable for either a history of engaging in maladaptive compensatory strategies or for "conditioned arousal" itself.

If the insomnia is chronic (>1–6 months), it is overwhelmingly likely that (1) the patient has engaged in the kind of compensatory strategies that are targeted with CBT-I, and/or (2) enough time has passed so that the insomnia is now a conditioned phenomena. That is, the repeated pairing of sleep-related stimuli with wakefulness and arousal is thought to produce a conditioned cognitive, somatic, and/or central nervous system form of arousal (55;56) which persists regardless of the original precipitating or perpetuating factors (maladaptive compensatory strategies).

If the insomnia is transient (<1–6 months), this suggests that the precipitating factors may be responsible for the insomnia. As noted below, the precipitating factors may be acute medical or mental illness and these factors may serve as contraindications for CBT-I. On the other hand, a good clinical interview and/or a contingency analysis may reveal that (1) psychosocial factors are driving the insomnia and may require an intervention but probably not CBT-I, or (2) the patient has recently begun engaging in the compensatory strategies which undermine good sleep continuity and accordingly may be ideal for an early intervention.

- *Is there evidence that the insomnia is maintained by "conditioned arousal?"*

During the clinical interview one can acquire evidence that the conditioned arousal exists, and often with two standard interview questions.

First, when asked to describe the last hour of the day—for an average day—patients with primary insomnia often report being sleepy or falling asleep on the couch and then suddenly becoming awake when walking into the bedroom. While the patient may attribute this to walking too quickly, or to engaging in too many prebed rituals, this is thought to represent an elicited arousal; the eliciting stimuli being the bedroom, the bed, bedtime, and so on.

Second, when asked to describe how they sleep when in an alternate bedroom or when traveling, patients with primary insomnia may report that their sleep is improved. This is thought to occur because the novel sleep environment is relatively free of the normal eliciting stimuli. This may be a less reliable cue, however, because the conditioned arousal may not be limited to the individual's bedroom but also extend to the act of going to bed, bedtime, and so on. As result, the patient may sleep as poorly in novel environments as at home.

- *Is duration of sleep (TST) an important consideration?*

No. Any report regarding total sleep time is only meaningful if there is a daytime complaint. That is, for example, "I am only getting X hours of sleep per night and because of this I feel terrible during the day as if I have not slept enough . . ." What is important about this statement is, regardless of the value for *"X,"* is the consequences of *"X."* Thus, it can be argued that one need not define TST to know that CBT-I is indicated. All that one need know is that there are sleep continuity problems and daytime sequelae. In addition, what constitutes normal total sleep time is unknown and is thought to vary substantially from individual to individual.

The Contraindications for CBT-I

Having established that CBT-I *may be* indicated, the next step is to consider exclusionary criteria and/or to determine if CBT-I is contraindicated. Simply establishing the following benchmark can do this.

- *The patient has a medical or psychiatric illness which is undiagnosed, unstable, or may in and of itself interfere with CBT-I.*

Evidence for this may be gleaned from the clinic questionnaires, the clinical interview, and/or from direct interaction with the patient's primary care physician and/or psychiatrist. For a list of common factors that contribute to or complicate the treatment of insomnia, see Table 4.2.

When it is clear that the patient has an unresolved or unstable illness, the clinician may elect to defer treatment for one of three reasons.

TABLE 4.2. Common Factors That Contribute to or Complicate the Treatment of Insomnia

Medical illness
Head injuries, hyperthyroidism, chronic obstructive pulmonary disease, asthma, hypertension, coronary artery disease, arthritis, fibromyalgia, headache and low back pain, seizures, gastroesophageal reflux disorder, Parkinson's disease, Alzheimer's disease, diabetes, cancer, benign hypertrophic prostatitis, menopause, etc.

Psychiatric illness
Major depression, generalized anxiety disorder, posttraumatic stress disorder, panic disorder, bipolar disorder, dementia, schizophrenia

Acute medication effects
Alcohol, amphetamines, caffeine, reserpine, clonidine, SSRI antidepressants, steroids, L-dopa, theophyline, nicotine, nifedipine, beta agonists (albuterol), etc.

Withdrawal medication effects
Benzodiazepines, barbiturates, alcohol

Other sleep disorders
Obstructive sleep apnea, narcolepsy, nocturnal myoclonus, restless legs syndrome, phase advance sleep disorder, phase delay sleep disorder, sleep state misperception disorder, nightmare disorder, parasomnias, etc.

Situational factors
Life-stress, bereavement, unfamiliar sleep environment, jet lag, shiftwork

Source: Adapted from Diagnosis of Primary Insomnia and Treatment Options. Invited Paper to *Comprehensive Therapy* 2000; 26(4); 298–306.

First, it is suspected that the insomnia may resolve with the acute illness or once the illness is stabilized. If this is the case, it may be useful to inform the patient that the insomnia will likely clear up. In addition, the patient should be counseled to avoid engaging in compensatory strategies when experiencing acute episodes of insomnia. For further information regarding prophylactic strategies, see the section dedicated to relapse prevention (Session 8).

Second, it is suspected that the insomnia will not resolve but that the acute illness will prevent the patient from engaging in or benefiting from therapy. The patient may be unable to engage in therapy because she is not physically up to the tasks of sleep restriction or stimulus control (e.g., patients with acute illnesses that require increased sleep or increased time in bed, acute injuries that prevent the patient from walking, etc.). In this case, the patient should be told that effective treatment is available, but to maximize treatment outcome, therapy should be delayed. It may be helpful to assure the patient that help will be available at a later point in time and (if possible) that she/he will have expedited access to services.

Third, it is suspected that CBT-I will aggravate the acute illness. In many instances, the decision to delay treatment will be based more on clinical wisdom than the force of empirical data. For example, while it is suspected that febrile illnesses and/or infectious diseases require increased sleep for recovery, this is—at this time—strictly a clinical wisdom. This said, it is nonetheless wise to follow the standard of practice, and delay treatment for the insomnia.

In some cases, one need not take into consideration the above issues. There will be clear evidence that CBT-I is contraindicated. To make this determination, the question one must be prepared to answer (or to seek out consultation for) is—"will treatment lead to an exacerbation of the acute illness?" This is clearly a possibility for patients with epilepsy, bipolar illnesses, parasomnias, obstructive sleep apnea, or other illnesses that have excessive daytime sleepiness as a feature of the parent disorder. Sleep loss through sleep restriction may lower the threshold for seizures in epileptic patients, may precipitate mania in bipolar patients, may exacerbate parasomnias, may prevent adequate ventilation in patients with obstructive sleep apnea, and/or may simply aggravate day time somnolence (EDS) to a point where it is no longer safe for the patient to drive, operate machinery, and/or make judgments that adequately promote their own and/or the safety and well-being of others.

With respect to this last point, if EDS is present, combined therapy may be indicated (CBT-I + a wake-promoting substance like modafinil or methylphenidate). It should be noted, however, that there is only limited data with respect to this form of combined therapy (57). The data that exist suggest that modafinil (qam 100 mg) may be combined with CBT-I and, while diminishing daytime sleepiness, does not interfere with treatment outcome. For additional information on this form of combined therapy. (Perlis ML. Smith MT. Orff HJ. Enright T. Nowakowski S. Jungquist C. Plotkin K. The Effects of Modafinil and CBT on Sleep Continuity in Patients with Primary Insomnia. *Sleep* 2004;27(4) 715–725.)

Present an Overview of Treatment Options

Once it is clear that CBT-I is indicated, the patient needs to be presented with treatment options. In the clinical setting where pharmacotherapy is available, the clinician should review the "pros" and "cons" of the three possible strategies (CBT-I; pharmacotherapy with hypnotics; pharmacotherapy with sedating antidepressants) while taking into account the patient's treatment history. Reviewing the treatment options provides the patient the knowledge she/he needs to make informed decisions and the opportunity to have a say regarding their care. For example (with a treatment naïve patient):

Dialogue #3: Presentation of Treatment Options

Therapist: At this point, I think I have all the information I need. What I'd like to do is review your treatment options with you. Once we have done this, and I have answered your questions, I'm going to want you to defer treatment for one week so that you can decide which treatment you want to pursue and so we can collect some addi-

tional information with sleep diaries. But let's not get ahead of ourselves—let's take some time to review the options.

Option 1. Go on as you have been but with the knowledge that the insomnia is not likely a sign or symptom of something more serious. The up side here is that you don't have to engage in any form of treatment just now. The down side is that it is unlikely that the insomnia will, at this point, go away on its own.

Option 2. We can, in collaboration with our medical staff, have a prescription written for you for one of several types of sleeping pills. In our clinic we tend to work with two types of medications—one type are called benzodiazepines (for example temazepam) and the other type are called (for want of a better expression) nonbenzozodiazepines (for example zolpidem or zaleplon). Of the two, we tend to recommend medications like zolpidem or zaleplon because they tend to not interfere with the quality of your sleep and do not seem to have withdrawal effects. The up side with these meds is that they provide immediate relief and between 30% to 50% improvement, the gains appear to be stable for periods of up to 3 to 6 months, and the meds tend to promote a kind of sleep that appears to be relatively normal. The down side is that the meds do not "cure." That is, once you stop taking the medication, the best-case scenario is that you're back where you started.

Option 3. We can, in collaboration with our medical staff, have a prescription written for you for one of several types of antidepressants that are often prescribed to help people sleep. The up side with these meds is that they also provide immediate relief, the gains appear to be stable for long periods of time (6 months to years), and they also seem not to produce withdrawal symptoms. The down side is that these meds appear to have more limited effects on sleep onset problems, they produce smaller clinical gains, they alter sleep quality, and they may have unpleasant side effects. Whether these meds produce long-term gains after the meds are discontinued is unknown.

Option 4. We can treat your insomnia with cognitive behavioral therapy. This a nonpharmacological intervention that takes approximately 5 to 8 weeks to complete. The up side is that it's very well tested: it has been found to produce clinical gains that are comparable to (if not better than) sleeping pills, and the effects are long lasting. The down side is that it takes about 2 to 4 weeks for the intervention to begin to have an effect, you'll need to commit yourself to a process that takes between 5 and 8 sessions, and your insomnia will get worse before it gets better.

Please take some time to ask questions and then let's review what we need to do between now and next week.

Discontinue Sedative Hypnotic Medication Use

In many cases patients come into therapy using a variety of medications. Some will be using medications to help them sleep. Of these patients, some may wish to discontinue medication, while others are more hesitant to stop using sedatives. If the medication is prescribed for sleep, CBT-I is most likely to be successful if the medications are discontinued before treatment. A positive approach to this process is to collaborate with the prescribing physician and to phase in the withdrawal. Several investigators have developed withdrawal protocols (58;59).

The gradual withdrawal of medication serves several purposes. First, it maximizes the patient's safety during the withdrawal (e.g., rapid withdraw from benzodiazepines may result in seizures). Second, if data are collected during this period (e.g., 4 week protocol: Week 1, regular use of meds; Week 2, half the medication amount [either by day or amount]; Week 3, half again the medication amount; Week 4, no medication), it is likely that the data will show (1) that the negative effects of withdrawal, if they occur, are short lived and (2) minimal differences between regular use and no use of medication. Third, the withdrawal before therapy will prevent a setback because of patient withdrawal at a later time. For a list of hypnotic medications or medications that are used as sedatives, see Table 4.3.

TABLE 4.3. Medications

Trade name	Generic name	Class of medication	FDA indication	Dose (mq)	Ti$_{\max}$ min	½ life hrs
Ambien	Zolpidem	BZRAs	Insomnia	5–10	30–50	2.5–5.6
Sonata	Zaleplon	BZRAs	Insomnia	5–20	30–60	1–2
Estorra	Eszopiclone	BZRAs	Insomnia	1–3	1.0–1.5	4–6
***	Indipion-IR	BZRAs	Insomnia	10–20	50	1.5
***	Indipion-MR	BZRAs	Insomnia	10–20	60–120	1.5
Dalmane	Flurazepam	Benzodiazepine	Insomnia	15–30	30–60	47–100
Doral	Quazepam	Benzodiazepine	Insomnia	7.5–15	60–90	25–41
Magadan	Nitrazepam	Benzodiazepine	Insomnia	2.5–5.0	30–120	18–25
Prosom	Estazolam	Benzodiazepine	Insomnia	1–2	60–90	8–24
Restoril	Temazepam	Benzodiazepine	Insomnia	7.5–30	20–50	3.5–18
Halcion	Triazolam	Benzodiazepine	Insomnia	0.125–0.25	50–120	3–4
Xanax	Alprazolam	Benzodiazepine	Anxiety	0.25–0.5	60–120	9–20
Klonopin	Clonazepam	Benzodiazepine	Anxiety	0.5–2.0	60–240	19–60
Valium	Diazepam	Benzodiazepine	Anxiety	2–10	60–120	20–50
Ativan	Lorazepam	Benzodiazepine	Anxiety	0.5–2.0	120–240	8–24
Elavil	Amitriptyline	Tricyclic	Depression	25–150	2–8	5–45
Sinequan	Doxepin	Tricyclic	Depression	25–150	2–8	10–30
Desyrel	Trazodone	5HT agonist	Depression	25–150	3–14	3–10
Serzone	Nefazadone	5HT agonist	Depression	50–150	1	2–4
Seroquel	Quetiapine	Dibenzothrazepine	Antipsychotic	25–50	1.5	4–8
—	Chloral Hydrate	—	Sedation	50–1000	30–60	4–6
Benadryl	Diphenhydramine	Antihistamine	Allergy Relief	25–100	0.25–0.5	3–12

In some cases, patients will present on medications which are being prescribed for another problem but which have secondary benefits for their sleep (i.e. some antidepressant medications, klonopin for seizures or PLMS, etc.). In these cases, the patient will generally stay on the medication and treatment will proceed.

Dialogue #4: Should I Continue with My Current Medications While in Treatment?

Patient: My doctor thinks I should stay on my antidepressant for another six months at least to keep my depression in check. Is that okay?"

Therapist: This makes sense. So let's work on your sleep. If we're successful, this may even have some significant protective or prophylactic value regarding your depression and may make it more likely that in six months you can discontinue your antidepressant and stay well.

Orient Patient to the Sleep Diary

While most patients are familiar with the idea of keeping a diary or a daily log, the practice of doing so for evaluation purposes may be somewhat new. It is important to explain the purpose of the diary, highlighting that it (1) allows for "sampling" and provides more reliable estimates (i.e., that it is relatively free from memory heuristics like recency, saliency and primacy), (2) if need be, allows for the clinician to undertake contingency analyses, and (3) is the data source for therapy and allows for the formal assessment of treatment outcome, both for the individual and for the clinic as a whole.

It is critical to complete a diary *with the patient*. First, complete a day's worth based on "your" sleep and wakefulness data from the previous day. As part of this, it is critical to demonstrate that not all the variables on the sleep diary are "guesstimates." Sleep Latency (SL) and Wake After Sleep Onset (WASO) are based on only the patient's subjective impressions. This said, it is important to make sure that patients include time awake as a result of early morning awakenings with the WASO estimates. Time in Bed (TIB) and Total Sleep Time (TST) are calculated variables. TIB is calculated as minutes elapsed from "lights out" to "lights on." For example, if "lights out" is at 10 PM and "lights on" is at 5 AM, then TIB equals 420 minutes. TST is calculated as TIB − (SL + WASO). For example, if TIB was 420 minutes and SL was 30 minutes and WASO was 30 minutes (30 + 30 = 60 minutes), then TST equals 360 minutes. After providing an example, have the patient

complete a day's entry based on her experiences for the day before the clinic intake. If, after two examples are completed, the patient appears to continue to have trouble completing the form, consider engaging one or two more practice attempts with data you provide. If this continues to be a problem, consider using (if available) actigraphy.

At the close of the session, remind the patient to "sleep as usual." Emphasize that it is important that an accurate sample/baseline be obtained. Only one sleep-related behavior should be altered: have the patient turn the clock away from the bed and only check the time before going to bed and when getting out of bed in the morning to start the day. This provision is enacted so that the data collected during and after treatment will be parallel with that obtained during the baseline week. If actigraphs are being used, the patient should also remember to click the event marker button at "lights off" and at "lights on."

Field Patient Questions and Address Resistances

While there are an infinite number of questions and resistances that might arise at this point in therapy, the most common concern of patients pertains to the fact that treatment is not immediately forthcoming. Below is a sample dialogue addressing this issue.

Dialogue #5: Why Can't I Start Treatment Immediately?

Patient: Isn't there anything I can do between now and next week to improve my sleep?

Therapist: It is very important that you not only understand *what* steps to carry out but also *why* you are carrying them out. Today we will not have the time to cover all the steps and the rationale for those steps. Therefore, I would rather not give you incomplete lists of instructions. As important, the data we gather during the next week are critical for our getting an accurate picture of your sleep problem and they will serve to guide your treatment.

Maybe it'll help to think of it this way—let's say you were referred to a neurologist for severe headaches. Would it make sense for him to say, "oh you have headaches, they're most likely related to localized cortical ischemia, let's have you take this medication. . . ." Instead, wouldn't you prefer that she/he did some assessment work before starting treatment?

Patient: Absolutely. I wouldn't want to be taking medication just because my headaches are *most likely related* to something. I'd want her to be sure of the diagnosis before starting treatment.

Therapist: Same thing here. We need to know what we're dealing with. . . .

Patient: But can't you tell me just one thing that can help?

Therapist: As I said, we need to get a better assessment of your sleep problem before we start treatment. So we need to wait. But there are at least two other reasons we need to wait.

First, some of the things we're going to do are not obvious, and in some cases what we'll do is downright counterintuitive. We need to have the time to talk about these things and the time to make sure you understand the "why, where and when." Understanding will make it easier to do what you need to do. So I don't want to rush in before making make sure your 100% on board.

Second, if you carry out the "just one thing" incorrectly or the "one thing" doesn't produce much relief by itself, it will only produce more frustration and less willingness on your part to carry out that step when it is integrated into the whole program.

So . . . believe me when I tell you, it'll work much better to wait for a time when we can provide you not only with a list of steps but a basis for understanding why you will be carrying out the steps, how they will work, and how long it will take for them to work.

Setting the Weekly Agenda

Set the patient's expectation for the following session. Be sure to let her/him know that the first order of business for the next session (and all sessions that may follow) is to review the sleep diary data and to track the patient's progress in a systematic and data driven way.

Dialogue #6: Setting Expectations for Weekly Agenda

Therapist: Next week when you come in the first thing we do is review your sleep diary data. The plan will be for you to come through the door, sit down, and start reading numbers. My job will be to calculate your weekly averages and to begin a graph, which we will use to track your progress. I know it sounds kind of "mercenary" or excessively business like . . . but almost as important as having the data . . . is having your understanding that the kind of treatment we offer is based on the data you provide—that the treatment is "data driven." I know once we get into the swing of this, you'll appreciate the approach. Most folks do. So we'll see you next week, and if you have questions during the week, especially questions about the diary, feel free to call or drop me an E-mail.

Session Two: Treatment Initiation (60 to 120 Minutes)

> ## *Tasks*
>
> Summarize and Graph Sleep Diary
> Determine Treatment Plan
> Review Sleep Diary Data: "Mismatch"
> Introduce Behavioral Model of Insomnia
> Setting up Sleep Restriction and Stimulus Control
> Set Prescription (TIB and TOB)
> Set Strategy
>   How to Stay Awake to the Prescribed Hour
>   What to Do with WASO Time

Primary Goals of This Session

1. Review data and confirm that CBT-I is indicated
2. Select the treatment modality

If the patient opts for CBT-I:

3. Establish the rationale for the Sleep Restriction (SRT) and Stimulus Control (SCT)
4. Describe the approach to SRT and SCT and their efficacy, and provide an overview of the program.
5. Secure the patient's commitment to the program—one week at a time.

It should be noted in advance that this session is perhaps the most work intensive and difficult of the eight sessions because it requires an inordinate amount of teaching and persuasion. Considerable time is devoted to the effort to have patients conclude for themselves some of what might be presented didactically. Accordingly, much of this section is devoted to text explanations and to clinician–patient dialogue exemplars. With respect to the latter (and as indicated elsewhere in this book), these dialogues are not meant to be verbatim scripts (i.e., lines to be memorized), but rather examples of how one delivers the required information and the likely patient "counterpoints."

Summarize and Graph Sleep Diary

As with all in-office clinical contacts, this session begins with a review of the sleep diary. While the clinician can simply take the diary from the patient and "run" the averages, our sense is that this process is more collaborative by engaging the patient to read the data aloud. To promote a data focus, as opposed to a recap of one particular night, have the patient read the data for each sleep continuity parameter (row) as opposed to the

data across a given night (column). Averages should be calculated for sleep latency (SL), wake after sleep onset time (WASO), total sleep time (TST), and time in bed (TIB). In addition, sleep efficiency and average-time-to-bed (TTB) and time out of bed (TOB) should be calculated. In the case of the latter two variables, the easiest method for working with time variables is to translate them into measures of time elapsed from standardized anchors. For example, TTB may be represented as time elapsed in minutes from midnight (10 PM = −120, 3 AM = + 180 minutes) and TOB may be represented as time elapsed in minutes from 7 AM (10 AM = + 180, 3 AM = −240 minutes). The value of such an approach is that averages, deviations, and ranges can be calculated and the conversion back to clock time is relatively easy. Because, however, these calculations can be difficult for some patients, it may be best to leave the conversions for the clinician and make sure the diary has space for both clock time and "deviation time" (see Appendix 6).

Once the data is summarized, the clinician should graph the baseline values (see "Clinic Chart" in Chapter 3) and make the final judgment regarding the appropriateness of CBT-I for the patient. The first step in this process (as summarized in Figure 4.1) is to use the sleep diary data to determine if the presenting complaint is well suited to CBT-I. Thus, the initial questions to be answered are:

- On average, is the patient's SL or WASO greater than 30 minutes per night?
- On average, is the patient's SE% less than 90%?

Note that this judgment is not made based on the match between diagnosis and treatment but rather on the basis of the match between presenting symptoms and treatment. That is, does the patient exhibit the "maladaptive behaviors" (represented by low sleep efficiency) that are the "targets" for the behavioral component of CBT-I?

Provided that the patient is a good candidate for CBT-I, the next question is which of the three treatment modalities the patient prefers. In the previous session, the patient received information regarding all three approaches. Most patients will opt for CBT-I for one of two reasons. First, they have been treated with either hypnotics or sedative antidepressants and have experienced first hand that these may produce good short-term gains but have the risk of side effects, dependence, loss of efficacy, and the need for long-term use to maintain the clinical gains. Second, patients seem to have an intuitive sense that something other than the original precipitants are maintaining their insomnia and that CBT-I may allow them to finally "get at the cause" of the insomnia.

For the patient's that prefer medication, it is perhaps best to allow them this choice, at least for the short term. Requiring a patient who prefers medication to engage in CBT-I is likely to result in a poor treatment outcome given the level of patient collaboration that is required for a successful intervention. By allowing for this measure of "autonomy," the clinician opens the door to the possibility that the patient will freely choose CBT-I

at a later point in time. For the patient's who choose CBT-I, the first step is to use the patient's own data to demonstrate some of the principles that are fundamental to the behavioral perspective.

Review Sleep Diary Data—"Mismatch"

When reviewing the sleep diary with the patient, the calculation of average TST and TIB provides a unique opportunity to make the first of several critical points: that there is a mismatch between TST and TIB. This means that the patient is trading the possibility of more sleep for the likelihood that sleep will be hard to initiate and that it will be fragmented and shallow. It is also important to take this initial opportunity to draw attention to the patient's tendency to stay in bed when awake because she/he is "waiting for sleep" or because "lying in bed is at least restful."

Dialogue #7: Discussion of the "Mismatch" Between TIB and TST

Therapist: Over the course of the last week you averaged 5.5 hours of sleep per night. This said, there is clearly some variability around this average number. The variability may have occurred for any number of reasons ranging from

- how you slept on the prior night, to
- how much light exposure you had during the day, to
- what and when you ate, to
- whether you exercised during the day or showered at night, to
- how long you were continuously awake
- and so on.

What's clear is that, on average, you can "generate" 5.5 hours sleep. One way of thinking about this number is that it represents your "sleep ability." That is, the amount of sleep, on average, you can generate.

Also apparent from your sleep diary is that, at least for last week, you spent an average of 7 hours in bed.

Okay—Here's the question: if you can generate 5.5 hours of sleep, why are you spending 7 hours in bed?

Patient: If I spend more time in bed, I'll get more sleep.

Therapist: On average is this the case?

Patient: No, but sometimes this works.

Therapist: Okay. But a lot of the time it doesn't, because you still have a sleep problem. Right?

Patient: Right. But sometimes its better.

Therapist: Okay. But sometimes it's worse. You lie in bed upset by the fact that it's another sleepless night.

Patient: Sometimes. But sometimes it's restful. And isn't rest better than nothing?

Therapist: Let's look at it this way. When you stay in bed awake, a third of the time you get more sleep (by the by I doubt this, but for argument's sake I'll grant you this), a third of the time you at least "get some rest," and a third of the time you lie in bed annoyed or at least "unable to not think about stuff."

The bottom line here, given that sleep is what you are after, is that you are trading about 30% success rate for 70% failure. This sound like a good bet?

Patient: When you put it that way, I guess not.

Therapist: Okay. Lets take some time to talk about the consequences of "extending sleep opportunity" (that is staying in bed for longer periods of time in the hope that you'll get more sleep) and the consequences of "staying in bed" waiting for sleep.

Introduce the Behavioral Model of Insomnia

While there is no question that the model is of value to the clinician, it is important that it be shared with the patient. Presenting the perspective to the patient allows the clinician a means by which he/she may demonstrate how it is possible for insomnia to "have a life of its own." This will help the patient to understand why the interventions make sense and is likely to increase enhance adherence.

When presenting the behavioral model, the clinician should start from scratch and draw the model on a dry erase board (as opposed to providing a handout or using a slide presented on a computer screen). Drawing the model will slow the process and make it more accessible to the patient. Once the model is up on the board, the clinician should take the time to apply it to the individual case and use the platform as means for enabling the patient to deduce what behavioral interventions might be useful. The following dialogue should serve as an example of how the model can be used to introduce and "sell" sleep restriction therapy and stimulus control.

Dialogue #8: Discussion of Predisposing, Precipitating, and Perpetuating Factors

Therapist: Now that I've shared with you the general model, let's take some time to see how this applies to you. For the predisposing factors, it seems to me that there are a few things that might apply:

- Maybe some genetic predisposition given that your mother had a long-standing problem with insomnia.
- Maybe a biological predisposition given your tendency to be easy startled or physically tense.
- Maybe some psychological predisposition given your tendency to "mull things over" and to worry.
- Maybe some social predisposition given that you tend to go to bed earlier than you would otherwise, so that you and your spouse can go to bed at the same time.

As for the precipitating factors, it seems clear that going out on job interviews was very stressful for you and maybe that event accounts for how the insomnia began.

Finally, and most importantly, you seem to have engaged several of the behavioral factors we think are responsible for "perpetuating" insomnia. Can you name a few that apply?

Patient: You mean like going to bed earlier, getting out of bed later (whenever I can), staying in bed no matter what, and drinking like a fish to fall sleep at night?

Therapist: Those would be them. Let's spend some time with each of these, so that you might better understand that while these strategies seem like good ideas, they are at best short-term solutions with serious long-term consequences.

There is no question that when the insomnia is acute, going to bed earlier and/or getting out of bed later certainly allows one to recover some "lost sleep" and allows one to feel better during the following day.

The problem with the strategy is that sleep is, at least in part, homeostatically regulated. What this means is that there is a pressure that builds up while you are awake—a pressure for sleep. The longer you're awake, the more pressure there is for sleep on the night that follows. If you are already having problems falling asleep, going to bed earlier and/or getting out of bed later reduces the pressure for sleep on the following night. Thus, while you may feel better on the first night that you adopt this strategy, it is more likely that you will have problems falling asleep on the subsequent nights. It's not hard to see how this becomes a cycle. Sleep poorly, extend sleep opportunity. Extend sleep opportunity, sleep poorly.

But the cycle is not the only problem. What do you do when you can't sleep?

Patient: Stay in bed and try and sleep.

Therapist: Exactly. And both "staying in bed" and "trying to sleep" have negative consequences. It's a tough thing to will unconscious-

ness. Truth is, it's not possible, and the effort to do so is frustrating and annoying. Second, and perhaps most important, the repeated pairing of *being awake in bed* and *being frustrated and/or annoyed in bed* with the bed, bedroom, bedtime, and so on is a major problem.

Patient: How so?

Therapist: Let me put it this way. Describe the last hour of your day. Describe a typical evening.

Patient: Usually I fall asleep on the sofa, even when I'm trying to stay awake and watch TV, and then I make a "bee-line" for the bedroom. Sometimes I won't even brush my teeth because I'm afraid I'll miss the moment. I get into bed and nine times out ten, I'm wide awake.

Therapist: Right. And you're suddenly awake because . . . ?

Patient: Oh probably because I walked to the bedroom too quickly, or instead of trying to fall asleep, I started thinking about what I had to do the next day.

Therapist: I know it feels exactly like that, but maybe it doesn't have to do with walking too quickly, brushing, or not brushing your teeth. Maybe it's something else.

Patient: Like what?

Therapist: Hmmm. Let me think of an analogy. Okay. I am a single guy. Where do I eat dinner?

Patient: At restaurants.

Therapist: When I am at home, where do I eat my supper?

Patient: In front of the TV.

Therapist: Exactly. And on Sunday when I'm watching the big game, even after a big lunch, what do you imagine happens after I've been sitting in front of the tube for a while?

Patient: You feel hungry?

Therapist: Right. But its not about hunger; it's about repeatedly pairing hunger with watching TV. It's about something called classical conditioning. Can you see how this applies to your situation in which you spend large amounts of time in bed awake, in bed frustrated, in bed alert, and so on?

Patient: So you are saying that when I walk in the room and suddenly feel awake, it's like you're suddenly feeling hungry in front of the TV. You're saying this is an example of conditioning.

Therapist: Right. So here's where we find ourselves. We need to find a way to ensure that you fall asleep quickly and stay asleep for the duration of the night. We also need to make sure that when you are awake, you are not in the bed or bedroom. Let's consider each of these in turn.

Set Prescription

While the review of the behavioral model is a blend of the didactic and Socratic, setting the prescription can be done in either manner. Our bias is towards the Socratic, as we believe that the patient is more likely to adhere to rules that are not imperatives but rather "discovered" with their own internal logic (liberally but subtly guided by the clinician).

Dialogue #9: Setting up Sleep Restriction and Stimulus Control

Therapist: Before we spoke about the "pressure for sleep" and that you do things that, while well intentioned, diminish the pressure for sleep. What were these things, and what do you suspect we should do?

Patient: You're talking about my going to bed earlier, getting out of bed later. So I should stop doing this.

Therapist: Yes. But there is a way we approach this that is a bit more systematic, a way that takes into account your "sleep ability" and looks to "prime the sleep pump."

Here's what I mean. What time do you need to get up during the week to get to work on time?

Patient: 6:00 AM.

Therapist: Okay. 6:00 AM it is. Given that you, on average, sleep 5.5 hours per night and you need to be up at 6:00 AM, what time do you think we should set your bedtime if we want your sleep ability to match your sleep opportunity?

Patient: 12:30 AM.

Therapist: Right. But as we talked about earlier, we're not only dealing with the "mismatch" between what your body can produce and what you're asking of it, we're also dealing with conditioning, with a conditioned arousal. So what do you guess might happen for the first few nights when you've adopted this new sleep schedule?

Patient: I still might take a long time to fall asleep, so I am going to get less than 5.5 hours of sleep.

Therapist: Right. But in this instance, if you don't compensate in any way, what is likely to happen over the course of the week?

Patient: I'm going to be a train wreck.

Therapist: It's true that you may feel worse than usual during the day, and we need to talk about this and to plan for it, but for now let's stay with the night time consequences. After a few days of being very sleepy at bedtime, you should find it very easy to fall asleep, and this is our goal. Giving you the experience of falling asleep easily.

One more base to cover. What should you do when you find yourself in bed and unable to sleep? For that matter what do you normally do? You're lying there, you're annoyed, and you're wide-awake.

Patient: Sometimes I just stay in bed. You know, its warm, its comfortable. And then sometimes I get up and watch TV.

Therapist: Okay but while you are laying there, what are you hoping for?

Patient: That I fall back asleep.

Therapist: Right. And from your sleep diaries we see that, while you're hoping you're going to fall back asleep, you're in bed awake for an average of 45 minutes per night. Remember a few minutes ago when we talked about what happens when you walk into the bedroom after feeling sleepy on the couch?

Patient: Yes, I feel awake again.

Therapist: Yup. And that happens because. . . .

Patient: I've spent so many occasions being in bed awake.

Therapist: Right. So we want to avoid this scenario. We want to make sure that you're in the bed and bedroom only when you're very sleepy or asleep.

Patient: So when I wake up in the middle of the night the other strategy is better—get up and watch TV?

Therapist: Yup. Your instinct was and is a good one. But let me ask a question. When you start to feel sleepy on the couch, what do you do?

Patient: Usually sleep on the couch for a while. At least I can rack up a little sleep time on the couch.

Therapist: Right. But unfortunately this is sort of a missed opportunity, a missed opportunity to pair sleepiness and sleep with the bed and bedroom. Know what I mean?

Patient: But what happens is I wake myself back up if I try to make it to the bedroom.

Therapist: Yup. I know. We talked about this. So what do you think you need to do if this happens?

Patient: You're kidding? You want me to get up again and go back out to the couch?

Therapist: Right.

Patient: I'm going to be like a yo-yo the first couple of nights.

Therapist: Yup. But this is just a short-term thing and overtime if you continue to stay awake and out of bed, what should happen eventually?

Patient: I guess eventually I should become so sleepy that I will have to fall asleep when I get in bed.

Therapist: Right. So here is the rule of thumb: Every time you get in bed you are asleep quickly, or you are not in bed.

It is likely that the patient will offer resistance at this point. Resistance to stimulus control will often come in the form of an argument that "resting in bed is better than being fully awake." Careful attention needs to be paid to explaining why this is not necessarily the case.

Dialogue #10: Why Can't I at Least Rest in Bed?

Patient: Okay, I guess I get the stuff about conditioning, but I always thought that if I stayed in bed I was at least getting some rest. Isn't that a good thing to do?

Therapist: I'm glad that you brought that up. We think sleep has at least three functions. Two of those functions are relevant for the issue of whether "lying in bed is restful."

One is to conserve energy, and the other has something to do with repairing and rejuvenating the body. Let's say I grant you that lying in bed is as restful—is as conserving of energy—as sleep. Even if this were so—which I doubt—you're still setting up the circumstances for maladaptive conditioning (you know, pairing bed, bedroom, etc., with being awake, annoyed, etc.) AND you're missing out on the restorative aspects of sleep.

Patient: Maybe, but I was going to miss out on the restorative aspects anyway. So I might as well rest.

Therapist: Okay. Let's say you're willing to trade rest for the opportunity to "undo the insomnia." What kind of rest are we talking about? Leaving aside the half of the time that it's *really not restful* because you're upset and annoyed and focusing on the relatively rare moments where you feel "woozy and comfy," these may not have much value as "rest" either.

Let me ask a question. Are you willing to accept that when someone is anesthetized (both unconscious and immobile) that this must at least be as "restful" as laying in bed when one can't sleep?

Patient: I'd imagine so.

Therapist: Okay. Well there is an interesting body of research that shows that when sleep is replaced by anesthesia, the subjects, if allowed to sleep normally the following night, exhibit a form of sleep that looks as if they had been totally sleep deprived. This suggests that immobility and this form of unconsciousness is not a substitute for sleep and is apparently not very restful.

So, the far better bet is to forgo "the rest" and use the time when you can't sleep to work on undoing the insomnia.

Patient: I guess.

Therapist: I just inadvertently gave you an example of trading a short-term gain for a long-term gain. Let me now address this more explicitly. Let me draw a picture to show you what I mean for want of a better expression we refer to this as the clippers (see Figure 4.2).

Therapist: In the scenario we just talked about, resting represents this part of the curve. For arguments sake I'll grant you that you get some benefit from lying in bed and getting "rest." But as represented here in the curve, it's a short-term gain. In the long term, there is a cost. The cost is that the insomnia continues to be reinforced in the long term. Can you think of another example of something that fits on this side of "the equation."

Patient: Going to bed earlier after a bad night or two.

Therapist: Right. Why is this a trade-off?

Patient: I may fall asleep easily on that night, and that's great, but if what you say is true about there being a fixed amount of sleep I can get, then there's a possibility that I'm going to wake up in the middle of the night.

Therapist: Right.

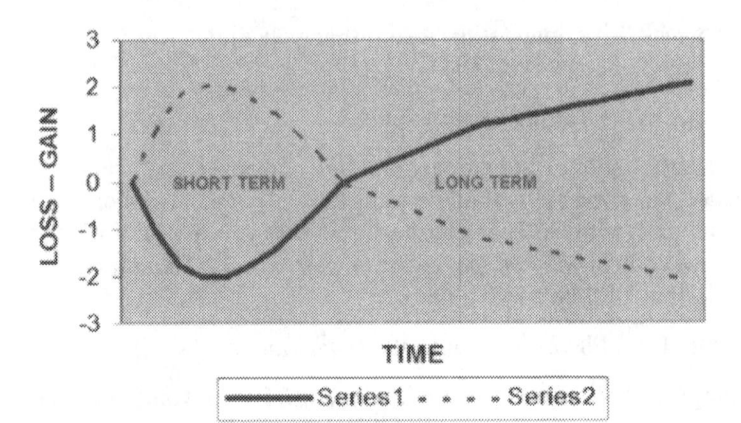

FIGURE 4.2. "Clippers."

Set Strategy

The primary goal is to make 100% certain that the patient understands the prescriptions and that a plan is enacted to provide for (1) activities while the patient is practicing sleep restriction and stimulus control and (2) the patient's concerns about fatigue and sleepiness levels during the first week or two of treatment.

Dialogue #11: Confirming Patient's Understanding of the "To-Do" List

Therapist: Now let's take some time and talk about how things need to work for the next little while, so we can "undo this insomnia" problem in the short term and set up the possibility of deconditioning it in the long term. What is it that I am asking you to do?

Patient: I need to go to bed at the same time every night. I need to get out of bed at the same time every day. If I'm having trouble falling sleep, or if I awaken in the middle of the night, I need to get out of bed.

Therapist: Right. So how are you going to know when to get out of bed?

Patient: Oh, maybe after half an hour?

Therapist: Nope. There is no rest for the weary. The moment you realize "I'm awake" or feel annoyed, you're out of there.

Patient: Doesn't this mean I'm going to end up with less sleep? I'll be a train wreck.

Therapist: Funny, you used exactly that expression last time. That is, if you really practice stimulus control as recommended, "you'll be a

train wreck." It's interesting to me that you didn't say you'll be "a plane wreck."

Patient: That's not the expression.

Therapist: I know. But I suspect that one reason we say "train wreck" versus "plane wreck" is that we want to imply "catastrophe," but one that is survivable. So I am glad to know that you feel that practicing stimulus control will just leave you "a train wreck." I'm guessing your feeling that "it'll be survivable."

Patient: Fine. I'll survive but in the short run.

Therapist: Yes in the short run it'll be hard. But it won't take long to get your body back on track. It's the clipper thing again. Short-term sacrifice for a long-term gain. What else do we need to be doing for the next while?

Patient: That sounds like everything to me.

Therapist: Almost. What time will you need to be going to bed and getting out of bed? And why?

Patient: I need to go to bed at 12:30 AM and get out of bed at 6:00 AM.

Therapist: Right and why? Isn't this going to mean that your get less sleep than normal, especially in the first few days? Why are we doing this ridiculous thing? I mean after all, you came in and said, "I can't fall asleep and stay asleep," and I am, in effect, saying, "So don't sleep" or rather "fine—sleep less." This is insane—no?

Patient: You bet it's insane, but you've been saying you want to "prime the pump." You want to use my insomnia to help me fall asleep quicker and stay asleep longer.

Therapist: Right. And if we're successful in pairing the bed and bedroom repeatedly with falling asleep quickly and staying asleep for "the duration." What do we believe will happen?

Patient: Eventually my insomnia will go away.

Therapist: Yup, the insomnia will be deconditioned.

Patient: Right. Fine. So I'm going to feel miserable during the day, and I'm going to be bored out of my mind at night, but this is okay because yada yada its the clipper thing, a short-term sacrifice for a long-term gain.

Therapist: Yup. But I'm not sure this has to be a suffer and sacrifice thing, at least not totally. So let's think of things that you can do at night when you can't sleep, things that are fun and that you enjoy. And for the next few weeks do these things, but only when you can't fall or stay asleep.

Real time should be spent developing a comprehensive list with the patient and reinforcing the notion that time spent awake should be a positive experience. There are at least two reasons for specifying that the experience should be a positive one. First, patients are more likely to engage in stimulus control practices if the exercise is somewhat enjoyable. Second, providing for positive experiences promotes a cognitive shift so that the patient's goal is changed from "trying to fall asleep or get back to sleep" to "how to enjoy their time while awake." This may also serve to diminish the anticipatory anxiety and/or derail the performance anxiety that is associated with sleep initiation or maintenance problems.

One way to help patients enjoy their time while awake is to identify a list of movies they have wanted to see or classics they enjoy. Armed with such a list, a week of rentals can be obtained for use "only at night." Whether movies, games, books, or hobbies, the important thing is to spend time in advance generating ideas rather than leaving it to the patient to do in the middle of the night.

Dialogue #12: What Happens If I Enjoy Staying Up Too Much?

Patient: What happens if I enjoy myself too much? Isn't there a chance that this could lead to more insomnia, like I might end up staying up the whole night!

Therapist: I am glad you asked this. It's possible that you could really get caught up in what you are doing and stay awake most of the night. But remember our plan is not to fix you tonight, but to bring about changes over the long term. So how well will you sleep the next night if you stick to the schedule?

Patient: I'll be exhausted but I guess sooner or later I'll sleep great, but I'll be a train wreck during the day. And I am not sure I can afford this.

Dealing with Excessive Daytime Sleepiness

Again, real time needs to be spent here. Is the patient concerned that she might be at risk for an accident and injury at work or on the way to work? Does the Epworth Sleepiness Scale data suggest that this person is at risk for true excessive daytime sleepiness? If so, the clinician should consider one of four possibilities. First, can the bulk of the initial sleep restriction (first 3–5 days of week 1) be done over a weekend or long weekend? Second, can the entire first week of sleep restriction be timed to correspond with a vacation or can the subject actually take some time off? Third, con-

sider sleep compression as an alternative to SRT. Fourth, is the patient a good candidate for stimulant therapy (modafinil, methylphenidate)? This approach has only been evaluated recently, but appears to be a promising way to manage this issue (57).

One drawback to accommodating the patient's concerns about the dire consequences of worsened sleep (by pretreating the emergent EDS, scheduling SRT to safe time, or altering therapy itself) is that this may undermine one of the subtler aspects of therapy. If the patient is allowed to make the conditions "safe," this eliminates the opportunity to evaluate the veracity of their fears that sleep loss will have catastrophic outcomes. Thus, leaving a seed of anxiety that treatment won't work in, or won't generalize to, real-world conditions. As important as this is, the clinician must balance between the benefit of this particular cognitive behavioral consideration and the patient's stated concerns and physical well-being.

One final point about the practice of sleep restriction. A plan needs to be enacted regarding how the patient will stay awake until the appointed hour (prescribed bedtime). As already exemplified in one of the dialogues, patients often nap on the couch during the last hour or two of the day. Such napping probably contributes to the patient's sleep onset problems (due the depriming of the sleep homeostat) and will certainly undercut the value of phase delaying bed time. The question for this session is whether the plan needs to be proactive or reactive. An argument can be made that it is better to determine, on the force of data, that such a problem exists rather than attempt to deal with this a priori. In either case, the clinician should be sure to monitor adherence so that this issue can be assessed prospectively.

One final point about the practice of stimulus control. While there is no prohibition against "getting too engaged while out of bed" there are several behaviors that one might engage in that may be counter-productive or fuel other problems. One such issue is related to light exposure. During the night even low level light may result in phase shifts (60,62), which may in turn exacerbate the insomnia or may even confer a new perpetuating factor to the primary disorder. Another issue is related to eating and drinking during the night. Eating should be avoided as it may reinforce your tendency to awaken during the night and/or may contribute to unwanted weight gain. Drinking to excess during the night, particularly alcohol, may lead to rebound insomnia, sleep inertia upon awakening (lack of alertness at awakening), and/or to problems with excessive alcohol consumption. Finally, exercise—while a good thing during the day—may at night lead to problems initiating or reinitiating sleep and that this may especially be the case when the exercise is engaged in with intent to "tucker one's self out."

Session Three: Sleep Titration and Sleep Hygiene (45–60 Minutes)

Tasks

Summarize and Graph Sleep Diary
Assess Treatment Gains and Compliance
Determine If Upward Titration Is Warranted
Review Sleep Hygiene

Primary Goals of This Session

1. Review data and confirm that upward titration is indicated
2. Assess treatment gains and compliance. In the case of noncompliance, focus session on this issue
3. Make adjustments to the patient's sleep schedule:
   - In the case of positive clinical gains (SE > 90%), upwardly titrate total sleep opportunity
   - In the case of no or marginal gains (SE between 85–90%), maintain schedule and provide rationale to the patient
   - In the case of negative gains (SE < 85%), downwardly titrate total sleep opportunity and provide rationale to the patient
4. Review sleep hygiene and tailor prescriptions to the individual
5. Continue to secure the patient's commitment to the program

Summarize and Graph Sleep Diary

As with all in-office clinical contacts, this session begins with a review of the sleep diary and the graphing of the weekly average values. Before calculating the weekly averages, the therapist should hand calculate each of the time in bed (TIB) and total sleep time (TST) values. This exercise is required to demonstrate that the patient is "keeping the books" according to "spec." Unfortunately, it is often the case that patients "guesstimate" all three of the standard sleep continuity variables, even though they have been coached to do otherwise. If this is the case, the beginning of this session needs to be strongly focused on the need to complete the diaries precisely as instructed.

Dialogue #13: Confirming TST Is Calculated and Not Estimated

Therapist: You may be wondering why I've gone to the trouble to "double check" your math. I've done this so that we can be sure that you're calculating TIB and TST accurately. In looking over your diaries, its clear that you took time and care in filling these out. The one thing that looks amiss is the total sleep values. Looks like you estimated these. In the future, remember that your total sleep time entries need to be consistent with your other entries.

Please remember that this is a calculated variable. Take the time to subtract both your sleep onset latency and the amount of time you are awake after sleep onset from the total time you are in bed to calculate your total sleep time. This way your TST will always be a reflection of these other numbers you estimated. Let's correct these numbers before we get on with the plan for today.

Once all the diary values are confirmed, weekly averages should be calculated. Two values are of primary importance: Sleep Efficiency and Total Sleep Time. If adult patients show a weekly average of <90% sleep efficiency (some allow elderly patients show <85% sleep efficiency), this suggests that there has not been an adequate response to sleep restriction and/or stimulus control therapy. This, along with the absence of a precipitous drop on the TST graph, provides evidence that the patient has not complied with the treatment recommendations. One way to more concretely assess for compliance is to use information from the sleep diaries to make a formal assessment of nonadherence.

Nonadherence

Sleep diary data may be used to calculate nonadherence given the known weekly prescriptions. This may be accomplished in a variety of ways (63). One way is based on the fact that since "time to bed" and "time out of bed" are prescribed and since there is a relatively absolute prohibition against spending time in bed awake or napping during the 8-week treatment interval, these parameters may be compared to that which is reported on the weekly diaries. In our hands this metric is compiled as deviations between the prescribed times and the reported times (in minutes). All the data needed is available from the sleep diaries provided that (1) the prescribed time to bed (PTTB) and prescribed time out of bed (PTOB) are recorded on this document and (2) one additional measure is added to the standard compliment: time out of bed (TOB).

For example, if the patient's "bedtime" is set at midnight and their "rise time" is set at 6 AM and the patient reported for a given day:

- went to bed at 11:30,
- a WASO of 60 minutes,
- a "time out of bed during the night" as 30 minutes,
- a rise time of 6:30 AM and napping for 30 minutes.

then the compliance measure would equal the sum the minutes deviate from prescribed time to equal 120 minutes of noncompliance for the given day. These values can, like the sleep continuity variables, be averaged to represent the mean noncompliance per week. There are no formal criteria for what constitutes non-compliance on this measure, but a "rule of thumb" might be equal to or more than 30 minutes per day.

If it is apparent from the sleep diary data that there were no significant clinical gains in the first treatment week, and there is evidence with the adherence measure that the patient did not comply to the sleep restriction therapy and/or stimulus control therapy regimens, then this issue supersedes all other considerations. The session needs to be entirely devoted to what factors prevented the patient from being adherent. The session must be devoted to either the effort to garner compliance or the decision to delay or discontinue treatment. Typically, nonadherence comes in one of three forms: the patient (1) wanted to but couldn't convince herself/himself to do it, (2) simply couldn't do it, and (3) didn't want to do it.

"Wanted to But Couldn't"

It is often the case that patients, when in session, agree wholeheartedly with the concepts, but often find that they "can't do what they should do" when they are attempting to delay their bedtime or attempting to leave the bedroom when awake during the night. As with addictions, a whole process of self-dissuasion seems to occur. For example:

"Not tonight we'll start tomorrow night."
"I really do feel sleepy, I know I should stay up, but maybe I should 'seize the moment' since I feel so sleepy."
"Its warm and comfortable in bed, if I get up the night chill will wake me up completely."

More cognitive work related to such thought processes is clearly indicated. One can revisit the issue of short- versus long-term gains (see Figure 4.2) or assail the derailing cognitions using a different heuristic.

Our approach to this form of nonadherence is based on the concept (and slogan) "it's a bad thing to be awake when reason sleeps." The concept, although not empirically validated, is that thought and impulse control are compromised during the nocturnal phase of the day. This may be so because the frontal lobe systems that are responsible for thought and impulse control are the first systems to go "off-line" (from a polysomnographic point of view), are the most compromised by fatigue and sleepiness, and may be the most subject to circadian variation. With respect to this last point, it may be the case that frontal lobe function is diminished during the night regard-

less of sleepiness, fatigue, and sleep deprivation considerations. Thus, patients may be unusually susceptible to "unreasonable logic" or "loss of reason based motivation" at the very time they need it most: when they're attempting to practice sleep restriction and stimulus control. Framing the problem of noncompliance in this way may have the value of enabling the patient to be more compliant because their nonadherence "wasn't their fault." Indeed, their noncompliance is understandable. If the patient goes into this situation knowing that there is a biological basis for being vulnerable to noncompliance, this may reenervate or reenable them to be more vigilant (i.e., to redouble their efforts against "self-dissuasion" ("I don't need to get out of bed because. . . .").

"Simply Couldn't"

In this instance, the patient also appears to have "bought the model," but does not report talking herself/himself out of following the required prescriptions. Instead, the patient reports that she/he simply could not stay awake until the appointed hour or arise from bed when awake during the night.

Given this scenario, it may be time for the therapist to carefully enact a plan to assist the patient with adherence. Several strategies are possible with respect to getting the patient to comply with the prescribed phase delay in bedtime (i.e., staying awake until the appointed hour). The possibilities include the following benign interventions:

• avoiding recumbent body positions during the last 1 to 3 hours of the night
• scheduled physical activity during the evening hours
• cold compresses to the extremities or small of the back.

More aggressive strategies, which require substantial caution and experience include:

• exposure to bright light during the evening hours
• careful use of caffeine during the evening hours
• use of stimulants (modafinil or methylphenidate).

These strategies, while potentially effective, run the risk of exacerbating the original problem or potentially creating new problems.

Getting the patient to adhere to the stimulus control component of therapy can be more challenging. Apart from the cognitive interventions (persuasion based on either the "clippers" or "sleep of reason" concepts) and the behavioral reinforcement strategy (engaging in enjoyable activities only during the practice of stimulus control) previously recommended, not much can be done to assist the patient with adherence to this aspect of treatment, the one exception being that morning use of stimulants may sufficiently block the negative consequences of stimulus control as to promote better adherence.

Another possibility is to consider evaluating to what extent sleep state misperception (subjective–objective discrepancy) is a feature of the presenting insomnia. This is important as it is possible that the baseline self-report measure of the patient's sleep continuity was more influenced by perceptual factors than "actual" sleep initiation or maintenance problems. If this is the case, curtailing the patient's sleep to their reported average may have resulted in more sleep loss than normally occurs with the acute application of SRT, thus leaving the patient so sleep deprived that they truly cannot stay awake until their prescribed time. If actigraphy was used during the baseline week, one can directly evaluate this issue. If actigraphy was not used during the baseline week, and is available, one might consider obtaining both sleep diary and actigraphic data during the second week. This will allow an assessment of whether there is a substantial discrepancy between reported TST and objectively measured TST.

"Didn't Want to"

In this instance, the patient simply has not "bought" the model, and the question for the clinician is "how likely is it that additional information and persuasion will be effective?" Our approach to this scenario is to be somewhat provocative; to simply let the patient know she/he is free to make her own decision and that one of those decisions is simply not to pursue treatment at this time.

Dialogue #14: Dealing with Noncompliance Using Cognitive Restructuring

Therapist: Okay. Here is where we find ourselves. At this point, you know the data as well as I. If you follow the regimen we have set out, you're likely to get between 30% to 50% better in the short term and still better than this in the long term. You know that what we're asking requires a trade off—"short-term pain for long-term gain." You seem to have made the judgment that short-term pain isn't worth it. You are certainly free to make this choice and if this is the way you want to go, we're done. Maybe this is the wrong time for us to be doing this work. But let me try one more time to put this in perspective. Tell me again, how long you have had your insomnia.

Patient: 5 years.

Therapist: Alright. Have you had the insomnia problem every night of those 5 years?

Patient: Probably not—more like 5 days a week.

Therapist: Okay. For argument's sake let's say 3 days a week. So if there are 52 weeks in a year (let's call it 50) and you have had insomnia 3 days a week, then you have had 150 nights of insomnia per year. This equals approximately 750 really miserable nights and days over the course of the last 5 years. Sound about right?

Patient: I guess.

Therapist: Okay. Remember the "clippers"? Well that's what we're talking about. I'm asking you to make a trade of 14–21 really bad nights to avoid another 750. Sounds like a good deal to me, but it's your choice. Shall we give this one more week or shall we opt to stop? And please know in advance, stopping is fine. It's your insomnia. If you want to keep it, it's yours to keep. So what's the choice; 14–21 for 750, or leave it be?

Alternatives to Nonadherence Issues

The last few paragraphs have been devoted to "nonadherence" issues. That is, the scenario where the subjects do not exhibit clinical gains and there is evidence of nonadherence. The alternative scenarios (all of which are based on the assumption or evidence that the patient has been compliant) are (1) the gains have meet expectation (≥90% sleep efficiency), (2) the gains have been marginal (between 85% and 90% sleep efficiency), or (3) there have been no clinical gains (<85%). Let us consider each of these in turn.

>90% Sleep Efficiency

This, of course, is the ideal. In this instance, the prescribed time to bed is phase advanced by 15 minutes, allowing for a potential upward titration of total sleep time by 15 minutes. This increment, standard to the Spielman approach, may seem unduly small to some patients (and to some clinicians as well). Presumably, the increment is optimal because there is less risk of a sudden reversal of gains. That is, in the event that the patient does not increase his/her total sleep time given an increase in total sleep opportunity (TSO), the reduction in the sleep efficiency quotient is less likely to fall below the level which constitutes reasonable sleep efficiency. For example, if the prescribed total sleep opportunity is 300 minutes and the patient is 90% sleep efficient (270 minutes) then an increase in TSO to 315 minutes without a corresponding increase in total sleep time (270 minutes) still yields an 85% sleep efficiency (270/315). Thus there is no reversal of gains and no need to downwardly titrate sleep opportunity.

Between 85% and 90% Sleep Efficiency

In this instance, the prescribed time to bed is unchanged, and there is no upward titration of total sleep time. The patient's prescribed time to bed

and sleep opportunity remain the same. The failure to achieve optimal gains in the first week of sleep restriction therapy should not necessarily be cause for alarm. Some patients require a larger accumulation of sleep debt for sleep consolidation. If the clinical course remains the same on the following week, a reevaluation may be needed. The issues to be considered at that time are related to the accuracy of the self report data (is the patient completing the diaries based on the facts or on what they think the clinician is looking for or wants to see?), the extent that so called sleep state misperception may be a factor, or that there is an occult medical, psychiatric, or substance use factor that is impeding forward progress.

<85% Sleep Efficiency

How this scenario is handled is somewhat controversial. According to the Spielman formulation of Sleep Restriction Therapy (SRT) (19), a sleep efficiency of less than 85% requires that sleep opportunity should be further curtailed by prescribing an additional phase delay of time to bed. In the original formulation, it is not clear whether this proceeds according to the "15-minute rule" or whether the new average total sleep time should be used to reset the prescribed time to bed. The algorithmic application of either strategy is likely to be effective, provided that the clinician is careful to avoid the scenario where the patient perceives the downward titration as "punishment."

Dialogue #15: What . . . I Have to Restrict Myself More?

Therapist: It seems as if the amount of sleep restriction that we prescribed has not been adequate to achieve the sleep efficiency that we are after. In my experience when I have seen this happen I have had good success with recalculating—recalibrating if you will—the sleep restriction.

Patient: I have a bad feeling that you are about to say something I don't want to hear.

Therapist: Right. I know the thought of restricting further at this time may feel difficult—like something you can't do or is the last thing you want to do. However, my concern is that if we leave you at this level of sleep restriction, we may go several weeks and not achieve our goals. In this case it will only prolong your suffering, potentially without any gain. If we restrict further at this time, it may cause you more discomfort in the short term but it stands a better chance of success in the longer run.

Patient: Yeah. The clippers. I know.

Therapist: Think of it this way. Think of dieting. If you eliminated some favorite foods from your diet (say ice cream and cookies) how would you feel?

Patient: Well I'd probably be missing those foods and maybe feel a little hungrier than usual.

Therapist: Okay. But how much weight do you think you would lose?

Patient: I've done that. You don't lose much.

Therapist: Right. So what do you have to do?

Patient: I hear you. I would have to put more effort into the process. Do it more systematically, like calorie count and calculate how much less I need to eat to produce weight loss. I'd be hungrier—for sure— but I'd get results and probably quicker.

Therapist: Right. Same idea here. We may have miscalculated the amount of calorie reduction required. After a week it's difficult to be sure.

So, the choice is yours.

We can keep things as they are, but in a week or two if we're in the same place, you can be sure that I'll recommend further sleep restriction. If we do this now, in a week or so we will be done with this part of treatment because either you will have begun to show good progress and we will be able to increase the amount of sleep you are getting, or we'll know for sure that another strategy is needed.

Review Sleep Hygiene and Tailor Prescriptions to the Individual

The first step of this intervention most often involves providing the patient with a handout. Following this, the various items are reviewed and the ratio-nales for each are provided. Table 3.1 contains a set of sleep hygiene instructions. It should be noted that in this formulation, several aspects of other therapies are adopted. For example, items 1, 2, 12, and 14 are tra-ditionally considered part of stimulus control and/or sleep restriction therapy.

Sleep hygiene education is most helpful when tailored to a behavioral analysis of the patient's sleep/wake behaviors. The tailoring process allows the clinician to (1) demonstrate the extent to which they comprehend the patient's individual circumstances (by knowing which items do and do not apply) and (2) critically review the rules, which are in many instances too "absolutistic." Let us consider two examples:

- The admonishment to avoid caffeinated products may be, in general, too simply construed. Caffeinated beverages may be used to combat daytime fatigue (especially during acute therapy) and, if the withdrawal is timed correctly, may actually enhance the subject's ability to fall asleep.
- The prohibition against napping may not be practical. Elderly subjects or subjects with extreme work performance demands may indeed need to compensate for sleep loss. A more considerate approach to napping may entail taking into account the time of the nap, the duration of the nap, and how nocturnal sleep is handled on days when subjects nap. Napping earlier in the day will allow for more homeostatic pressure for nocturnal sleep. Limiting the duration of the nap will allow for less of a discharge of the homeostat and enhance the subjects sensation of feeling rested from the nap (by avoiding awakening from slow wave sleep and suffering the ill effects of sleep inertia). Within limits, going to bed later, when one naps during the day, may minimize the effects of the nap on nocturnal sleep.

Finally, it can be argued that the most important aspect of sleep hygiene education derives not so much from the "tips" provided but from the exchange itself. A thoughtful and elaborate review may enhance the patient's confidence in her/his therapist and in the treatment regimen. Such enhanced confidence may, in turn, lead to greater adherence with the more difficult aspects of therapy.

An ideal procedure for administrating sleep hygiene is as follows:

1. Give the patient the list of rules and have her/him read them aloud and one at a time.
2. Review the "imperative" and explain the science behind the clinical practice.
3. Have the patient discuss how the rule applies to her/him.
4. Have the patient make a "to-do" list of items on the back of the handout (e.g., buy a set of new blankets, buy a new window treatments, etc.).

The therapist should keep a copy of the "to-do" list for use during the next session (i.e., review to determine if the items on the sleep hygiene "to-do" list were taken care of). Below we provide a prototype of a patient–clinician dialogue for each of the sleep hygiene items.

Dialogue #16: Sleep Hygiene #1, Homeostat, Wake Time, and Exercise

Patient: 1. Sleep only as much as you need to feel refreshed during the following day.

Therapist: Remember during our first session we talked about priming the homeostat? Well this is exactly what the first rule means.

Sleep restriction is all about consolidating your sleep by increasing your wakefulness and decreasing your time in bed. After the first few weeks of sleep restriction, you should feel more rested and actually be spending less time in bed.

Patient: 2. Get up the same time each day, 7 days a week.

Therapist: In some very real sense this is a training issue. Your body is being trained, is learning, when to be asleep and when to be awake. Reliably going to sleep and awakening to an alarm on a fixed schedule is likely to have conditioning effects so that, with time, your body will "on cue" know when to wake and when to sleep.

Patient: Am I going to have to do this forever? Does this mean that I'll have to use an alarm everyday and never get to sleep in on the weekends—never again?

Therapist: Yes and No. As I said, it's a training issue. While you're in training, it's a strict regimen. Once you're trained, things can be loosened up.

Patient: How long is the training?

Therapist: There's the 6 to 8 weeks that you "train" with me, but I'd be conservative and stay to a schedule for say 1 to 3 months. And when you do choose to start "sleeping in" on the weekends, you can (if you maintain the gains you've made during treatment), provided that you "play the game." If you want to sleep in an hour, okay but you should delay bedtime on the following night by an hour. This way you keep the amount of "pressure" for sleep constant. One thing: You may want to consider being careful about sudden and large changes to your sleep schedule. Maybe work up to sleeping in an hour on the weekends over 4 weekends where each weekend you add 15 minutes to your wake up time.

So, in the long run, you'll probably be able to "sleep in" on the weekends, provided you follow the plan. But lets talk about the alarm clock. In this instance, you'll probably want and need to use an alarm on a permanent basis.

Here's the reason. Lots of folks don't bother setting an alarm because they know they'll be awake in time to start their day. For folks who sleep well or who are happy with their sleep patterns, this is probably okay. For folks with insomnia, not using an alarm clock is a problem. This is true for patients with middle or late night insomnia, because it gives an adaptive function to the disorder. Put differently, giving the insomnia a purpose (any purpose) will make it harder to get rid of "because the insomnia is not entirely a bad thing—at least it gets me up in the morning." Using an alarm clock makes certain that the insomnia will not ever serve that purpose.

Patient: 3. Exercise regularly.

Therapist: Exercise is known to alter the nature of sleep. While its unclear whether daily exercise will cause one to fall asleep more quickly or stay asleep longer (in fact, the evidence to date looks like exercise is not helpful in this way), it is clear that "sleep architecture" is changed. Basically, exercise appears to hasten how quickly one descends into deep sleep (stages 3 and 4) and promotes more intense and/or larger amounts of deep sleep. Both probably good things.

This might be an ideal place to draw a hypnogram on the dry erase board and talk about sleep stages and the characteristics and putative functions of the various sleep stages. Such a demonstration is likely to be interesting and will provide the patient an increased understanding of the factors related to her/his insomnia which should, in turn, have the effect of enhancing compliance.

Dialogue #17: Sleep Hygiene #2, Exercise Alternatives and Bedroom Environment

Therapist: Interestingly, it may not be the exercise per se, but rather the change in body temperature that occurs with exercise. The idea is that when body temperature is increased, the cooling off that occurs when one lies down to go to sleep occurs in a more radical fashion, and it is this phenomena that has something to do with the promotion of slow wave sleep. Given this idea, how else might you increase your body temperature without exercise?

Patient: A hot bath or sitting in a hot tub?

Therapist: Yup. There have been a series of studies that show that a reasonably hot bath 1.5 to 2 hours before bed has many of the same sleep effects as aerobic exercise. Plus, having a prebed ritual is good thing—in part for the cuing thing we talked about a few minutes ago. And in part giving yourself some time to decompress and "put the day to sleep" is likely to help you to fall sleep.

Patient: 4. Make sure your bedroom is comfortable and free from light and noise.

Therapist: There are a couple of issues here. The first of which is probably people's expectation that low level noise or light *should not* keep them from falling asleep or cause awakenings. Well this may be true in one's teens and twenties, it is unfortunately the case that as

one gets older these things may be profoundly disruptive to sleep. And frankly, even in the instances where people report that such things aren't a problem, they have more of an effect than they may be aware.

Take, for example, people who live near airports. A PSG study looking at brain activity was done on such folks, and it was found that, even while most people reported that they didn't notice the overhead flights, every time a plane passed by there was an EEG arousal. This kind of arousal, by the by, is profoundly associated with daytime sleepiness and fatigue.

So the moral of the story is . . . ?

Patient: Go home and make sure my bedroom is better sound and light proofed.

Therapist: Right. Go home and do an assessment.

At sun up is the room pitch dark? If not, maybe new "window treatments" are in order. With the window closed, can you easily hear road noise or your neighbors? If so, you may want to consider increasing the amount of insulation in the wall, double pane windows, double thickness drywall, and so on. Most of these options are admittedly time intensive, if not down right expensive, but are well worth the time and expense.

Patient: How about the white noise generator or one of those sleep sound generators you see in in-flight catalogs that play whale sounds or ocean noise?

Therapist: Remember the airport study? Noise is noise, and its better to eliminate the occurrence of sound in your sleep environment. But if now isn't the time to be renovating the house, a sound generator is okay so long as whatever sound it generates is monotonous. So the whale sound is probably out, ocean sound is okay, but probably white or so-called "pink" noises are best. By the way there are companies out there that sell white noise forms of soothing sounds, and this may be the best compromise between a pleasing sound and the need for it to be invariant.

Patient: 5. Make sure that your bedroom is a comfortable temperature during the night.

Therapist: The general rule of thumb is any extreme in temperature is disruptive to sleep. This is so obvious that you don't need me to tell you. What may be less obvious is that, to say it in the vernacular, "sleep loves the cold."

As we may have spoken about on other occasions, body temperature varies over a 24-hour day and most people's preferred sleep

period occurs during the time of day when our body temperature is lowest.

Assuming there is a causal relationship here, and there is some data to suggest this is so, sleeping in a cool environment is likely to help one sleep. This said, it is important that one not be too cold. The simple remedy here is keep the room cold (60–68 degrees) and to layer on blankets. Having more blankets than you think you may need is a good idea because some stages of sleep require that you be more protected from ambient temperature than others.

Depending on how pressed for time one is, talking about the poikilothermia of REM sleep tends to be of interest to most patients. For clinician's unfamiliar with this phenomena, the basics are as follows. Thermoregulation is disrupted, if not entirely halted, during REM sleep. This is true in a variety of ways. Thermogenesis is halted because the sudden and global loss of skeletal muscle tension (1) interferes with the tonic production of heat and (2) prevents the shiver response to hypothermia. It is also the case that the ability to dissipate heat is impaired owing to peripheral vasoconstriction (prevents radiative cooling) and the inhibition of the sweat response (evaporative cooling). The inability to themoregulate during REM sleep along with the fact that the "on switches" for REM sleep are in primitive parts of the brain, has led some investigators to posit that REM sleep is phylogenetically older and to characterize the form of sleep as "reptile sleep."

Dialogue #18: Sleep Hygiene #3, Regular Meals, Fluid Restriction, and Caffeine

Patient: 6. Eat regular meals and do not go to bed hungry.

Therapist: Hunger may disturb sleep. A light snack at bedtime, especially carbohydrate, may help sleep, but avoid greasy or heavy foods that could initiate gastric reflux and cause middle of the night awakenings.

Patient: 7. Avoid excessive fluids in the evening.

Therapist: Reducing evening fluids can minimize nighttime awakenings. Here's a rule of thumb: stay within 1 cup of liquid (1/2 can of soda) within 4 hours of bedtime.

Patient: 8. Cut down on all caffeine products.

Therapist: While this may seem to be the most true of the various "sleep commandments," it is perhaps the least true and is, to my way

of thinking, "over-observed." It is often the case that people who have insomnia eliminate caffeinated products from their diet or routine. This may be a mistake. Like most things in life it's a matter of "how much and when."

It seems to me that a more productive approach is one that attempts to use caffeine in a therapeutic way. Coffee, for example, in the morning may substantially help to combat the ill effects of a poor nights sleep. Coffee, in the afternoon, may be used to combat the natural tendency towards "afternoon" fatigue, a thing that may or may not be exaggerated with insomnia. Coffee in the early evening may help enable one to stay awake to a later time. The combination of the latter two, may help increase the "pressure for sleep." Finally if timed just right, the caffeine withdrawal may help people feel sleepy at a time where they typically find it difficult to fall sleep. The trick is to find how much is enough and when to stop. This is, of course, not an easy thing to do. It depends on your sensitivity (prior use history), your body's metabolism, the kind of caffeine, and your willingness to find out by trial and error what works for you.

Here are some rules of thumb that may be especially useful during the course of treatment with us:

- If the clinical effects of caffeine last 4 to 6 hours (with a chemical half-life of 8–14 hours), then your last consumption should be 4 to 6 hours before your desired or prescribed bedtime.
- If you elect to use caffeine throughout the day, especially if you are not a regular coffee or tea drinker, be conservative about the number of times and the amount per occasion.
- Be prepared to limit or increase the amount of your intake, but do not make such adjustments on a day-to-day basis. Best to gather weekly data and make adjustments based on weekly averages for how you feel during the day and how you sleep at night.
- Finally, caffeine should be avoided entirely if you are prone to anxiety or have a medical reason not to be using caffeine.

If caffeine is going to be included for its therapeutic potential, the therapist would be wise to add a row to the sleep diary, so that the effects of this intervention can be monitored and regulated.

Dialogue #19: Sleep Hygiene #4, Alcohol and Nicotine

Patient: 9. Avoid alcohol, especially in the evening.

Therapist: Like the story with caffeine, this issue is also more complicated than the average person would have one believe.

Alcohol is the world's best and worst sleeping pill. For folks who have trouble winding down at the end of the day or who find themselves prone to being aggravated, upset, or moody in the evenings, alcohol does the trick. It promotes relaxation and has real anxiolytic properties (gets rid of anxiety) and it may even directly promote sleep given its CNS effects.

BUT—

"what alcohol giveth, it also taketh away." It has a relatively short half-life, which results in rebound arousal and rebound insomnia, and may be sufficiently dehydrating that this alone may promote awakenings. Bottom line: Modest amounts of alcohol may be useful to promote relaxation and to facilitate falling asleep. Drinking to promote sleep is likely to produce a trade off. One may fall asleep easily but end up reliably having early morning awakenings.

Let's take some time now review how much alcohol you are using and whether or not you might be using it as a hypnotic. But before we gather some info here, I need you to understand that my interest in your alcohol use is strictly limited to its effects on your sleep. Once I know this I can make recommendations regarding what changes you might want to consider. Whether you choose to do this is 100% your call. The main thing is that we know how much a factor this is and how it may be interfering with your sleep so that you make a informed choice.

NOTE: There are occasions where the clinician is genuinely concerned that alcohol use is leading to middle or terminal awakenings. In these instances, the clinician may wish to take a stronger position. This may be accomplished by having the patient refrain or decrease alcohol use for a week or two so that the effects on sleep continuity can be empirically assessed.

Patient: 10. Avoid smoking, especially during the night.

Therapist: Same story third verse. On the one hand, nicotine is a stimulant. Using stimulants when your trying to sleep is going to have a predictable effect—it's going to be hard to fall asleep. On the other hand, withdrawing from nicotine—especially for heavy smokers—may produce more physiologic arousal than satiating the need. The bottom line is

- Smoking above your usual level of consumption will have deleterious effects on your sleep.
- Smoking below your usual level of consumption will have deleterious effects on your sleep.
- Smoking when you usually don't (like in the middle of the night to "kill time") will have deleterious effects on your sleep.

Sound like a lose-lose scenario? It is, but the main issue for us is to determine if your middle of the night awakenings are being precipitated by nicotine withdraw.

For both alcohol and nicotine, the retrospective assessment of the patient's intake behaviors at the initial interview may have raised some concerns regarding the importance of these factors. If one is fortunate enough to have this be the case, one can initiate a contingency analysis during the baseline week by adding additional items to the sleep diaries. Such an assessment will allow the clinician and the patient the ability to determine if there is an association between the use of, or withdrawal from, these substances and the occurrence of middle or terminal insomnia. Unfortunately, it is often the case that substance use information only gets veridically reported later in treatment. Thus, the contingency analyses get deployed when the patient is partially treated and thus may result in vastly underestimating the importance of alcohol and nicotine as moderating factors. One indication that these factors may be "in play" is that the patient shows initial gains with sleep restriction, which diminish with time and the upward titration total sleep time.

Dialogue #20: Sleep Hygiene #5, Don't Take Problems to Bed

Patient: 11. Don't take your problems to bed.

Therapist: This sounds unbelievably obvious, but let's talk about it because there are two things I can tell you that make this a more interesting issue than first meets the eye.

First, as you know, sleep is not a unitary state: a thing you sink into, stay in, and then arise from 6 to 8 hours later. Instead there are at least 5 substages, creatively named Stage 1, Stage 2, Stage 3, Stage 4, and REM sleep. Collectively stages 1 to 4 are referred to as "non-REM." REM sleep, which I'm sure you have heard of, is indeed associated with dreaming. But what you may not know is that most people wake up briefly following REM sleep for some 10 to 90 seconds on each occasion. In people who sleep well, these awakenings may not be experienced as awakenings at the time, and are often not remembered at all in the morning.

But herein lies the rub: REM sleep is an intensely brain activated state and the awakenings that follow can also be characterized by intense brain activation. So one way of thinking about this is there are 4 to 5 occasions over the course of the night where your brain has the opportunity to "pick up the thread of wakefulness." If you take "your problems to bed," you have 4 to 5 occasions to be greeted by them during the night. As we have said before, don't give your insomnia a function (a time to problem solve).

The *second* interesting issue is whether it's worth even trying to think through your problems at night. There is a line of research we're interested in developing that we refer to as chrononeuropsychology. That's a really big word to say that we think that cognitive function varies drastically depending upon time of day.

The main idea is that during the night (the nocturnal phase of the 24-hour day), it is likely the case that most people are "cognitively impaired," but don't know it. We think that is has to do with the fact that the brain doesn't fall asleep all at once and that some parts of the brain fall asleep before other parts and/or more or less stay asleep even when the rest of the brain is awake. The part of the brain that is most likely asleep in the middle of the night has a lot to do with focusing your attention, logical thought, and the assessment of what is reasonable and not reasonable thought and behavior. With these functions compromised (in a way that is a lot like having had a bit too much too drink) its easy to see how one might all too easily make the jump from problem solving to just plain useless worrying. Given this point of view, you can see this is another reason to leave "thinking about stuff" to the day.

Bottom line: When you lay down to go to sleep or when you awaken the middle of the night, don't problem-solve or worry in bed. One simple way to defuse this situation, is make a list *before you go to bed* of the things you need to attend to the next day. If you wake up still thinking about these things, get out of bed and make a few notes. When you feel convinced that you've put enough of your thoughts on paper so that you can "pick up the thread" in the morning, go back to bed.

Earlier in this chapter, as part of the discussion regarding compliance ("Wanted to But Couldn't"), we introduced the concept of "it's a bad thing to be awake when reason sleeps." Here we have revisited the concept as it is applied to the middle of the night awakenings and the vulnerability to worry. Please remember that, at this time, these ideas are clinical truths. They have some value as aides to CBT-I, but await formal demonstrations regarding their veracity.

A lot more can be said here. For example, one might explain the idea of cognitive relaxation. Alternatively, one might spell out the idea that one can enter into a vicious cycle of worry, arousal and the inability to fall asleep, when mulling over important life issues in bed. The amount of time and manner of explanation regarding this important sleep hygiene instruction will, of course, vary with the therapists clinical orientation.

Dialogue #21: Sleep Hygiene #6, Don't Try to Fall Asleep

Patient: 12. Do not try to fall asleep.

Therapist: This is an important issue, one that is surprisingly obvious and yet not obvious. On the one hand, it's obvious that you simply cannot command yourself (or will yourself) to be relaxed and at peace and, even more obvious, you simply cannot command yourself to be "unconscious." Yet ironically, I hear this expression all the time: "I was trying to fall asleep and. . . ." Here's the irony, the mere act of trying is incompatible with what one is trying to do. You cannot be relaxed and exerting effort at the same time. You cannot unfocus your thoughts and disengage, when your thoughts are focused and you are indeed engaged in a task—"trying."

Sleep cannot be commanded or willed and despite the fact that we all know this, we "try to fall asleep."

Here's where some perspective may help.

Here's a silly but true analogy.

Sleep is like surfing. You can prepare to go surfing, you can have all the right equipment, but in the end, all you can do is paddle out and wait for the wave. You cannot will the wave to come; you can just be there when it does. In some ways, that is what sleep hygiene is all about, being prepared to surf when the wave comes in.

If the patient enjoys this analogy, one can spend some time with it, unpacking the potential similes. The wave is . . . ? The surfboard is . . . ? Your swimsuit is . . . ? The best time to surf is . . . ? And this is equivalent to . . . ? The person sitting on the board willing a wave to come is . . . ? But whether one unpacks the simile or not, it is important to get the patient on board with the idea that one can only optimize the likelihood of sleep, it cannot be forced.

Dialogue #22: Sleep Hygiene #7, Clock Watching and Naps

Patient: 13. Put the clock under the bed or turn it so that you cannot see it.

Therapist: If the alarm is set, there's no need to know in the middle of the night what time it is. That and, more importantly, clock watching can only lead to worry and frustration and if nothing else worry and frustration are "wind to the flame" of insomnia.

Patient: 14. Avoid naps.

Therapist: While most folks with insomnia don't or can't nap, so this may seem a nonissue, napping is an important thing for us to consider. It may become an issue during and after therapy.

Most people with insomnia experience intense fatigue (physical or mental weariness), but not the kind of sleepiness that allows them to nap during the day. During the first few weeks of therapy this may change. You may find that you want to, and can, nap.

There are two schools of thought on this. One suggests that napping should be avoided. The other allows for napping provided that certain "rules" are followed. Both schools of thought adhere to the idea that, at least in the short run, each individual can generate a fixed amount of sleep. So, if one naps during the day, there is less sleep available for the night.

Think of it this way. If you had a bank account and each day there's a deposit for $6 and each day you have $6 of expenses. What happens on the evening following a daytime withdrawal of a dollar?

Patient: I won't have the $6 I need in the evening but instead only $5.

Therapist: Right. So what do you do so you won't overdraw your account.

Patient: Only withdraw $5 on the days that I spend the $1 during the day.

Therapist: Yup. And this exactly one of the schools of thought. If your going to nap during the day then you adjust accordingly that night. Practically speaking, this means you delay your bed time by the amount of time you slept during the day.

There are two other rules of thumb here. First, short naps interfere less with the regulation of nighttime sleep. So it's best to sleep less than an hour, and probably best to sleep about half an hour if you want to stack the odds that you'll wake up from the nap feeling reasonably refreshed. Second, sleeping earlier in the day will interfere less with the regulation of nighttime sleep.

Patient: This seems pretty complicated. Maybe in the short run its best just not to nap.

Therapist: Right. That's the other school of thought. During therapy, don't nap.

Please remember that if you start feeling very sleepy during the day such that you feel that you are at risk for falling asleep at inappropriate times or places, that this is a serious issue and we need to address this.

Upon completing the sleep hygiene instructions, the clinician should summarize tasks for the week, make a copy of the patient's list of sleep hygiene tasks and introduce the concept that the next 1 to 3 sessions will be shorter visits that are primarily dedicated to sleep titration.

One final point with respect to sleep hygiene and the sleep environment. Remarkably, very little formal research has been conducted on sleep surfaces and/or on the effects of altering the home sleep environment. In the absence of hard data, "investing" in one's sleep environment (new mattress, pillows, bedroom furniture, wall colors, and/or lightening, and so on) may, at very least, have the effect of increasing the patients "stake" in the process of change. Beyond this, it also seems likely that significant alterations to the sleep environment may diminish the negative associations that exist vis-à-vis the bedroom and may promote improved sleep by weakening the "power" of the bedroom environment to elicit conditioned arousal. Finally, careful selection of a new mattress and pillows may promote improved sleep by diminishing orthopedic discomfort and/or pain.

Session Four: Sleep Titration (30 to 60 Minutes)

Tasks

Summarize and Graph Sleep Diary
Assess Treatment Gains and Compliance
Determine if Upward Titration Is Warranted

Primary Goals of This Session

1. Review data
2. Assess treatment gains and compliance. In the case of noncompliance, focus the session on this issue.
3. Make adjustments to the patient's sleep schedule
   - In the case of positive clinical gains (SE > 90%), upwardly titrate total sleep opportunity
   - In the case of no or marginal gains (SE between 85 and 90%), maintain schedule and provide rationale to the patient
   - In the case of negative gains (SE < 85%), downwardly titrate total sleep opportunity and provide rationale to the patient
4. Continue to secure the patient's commitment to the program.

Summarize and Graph Sleep Diary

As with all in-office clinical contacts, this session begins with a review of the sleep diary and the graphing of the weekly average values. Averages should be calculated and compared to previous weeks.

Assess Treatment Gains and Compliance

The primary question for this session is, at this point (if not before), has the patient begun to show signs of a clinical response. That is, do the adult patients show a weekly average of >90% sleep efficiency (or in the case of the elderly show a SE% of >85%) and does the TST graph show a precipitous drop?

If yes, the session should be focused on

- the upward titration of TST,
- a review of the sleep hygiene issues that were to be addressed as "homework."
- a review of strategies that help the patient be adequately alert during the day.
- a of review of strategies that help the patient stay awake to the appointed hour.

- a of review of strategies that help the patient practice good "stimulus control."

If there are not positive clinical gains and there is sleep diary evidence that the patient has not been adherent, then the clinician needs to reassess which form of noncompliance is at play. In the instances where the patient *"simply couldn't"* comply or *"wanted to but couldn't"* comply, the clinician needs to assess what it is that the patient "could not do." In most instances, the "couldn't" refers either to the patient's inability to stay awake to the appointed hour or the patient's inability to get out of bed in the middle of the night.

Evening bright light, afternoon caffeine, or morning (or split dose) modafinil may be used increase the patient's total wake time during the diurnal phase. Additional cognitive therapy may help with gaining compliance with the effort to practice stimulus control. One additional maneuver that may also be of use is to have patients "call in" to an answering machine in the middle of the night and encourage them to express their feelings about the practice of stimulus control at that moment (and that you as the therapist promise to listen to every "virulent" word).

In the instances where the patient persists with the fact that they simply *"didn't want to"* comply, one may wish to assess further for the factors that may be preventing compliance. For example, the apathy that may be associated with depression. This continued effort to secure compliance and treatment gains highlights that the assessment process is an ongoing endeavor. In fact, it is possible that, in this context, the patient may share information that was withheld or come to realize was more important than was previously apparent. Alternatively, it may be best to discourage the patient from continuing to let him/her know that you will be available at such a time as he/she is more ready to give treatment "a fair shot." When such an offer is coupled with the guarantee of expedited access to services in the future, this helps to show that the recommendation to discontinue services is not intended to be punitive.

Finally, if there are no clinical gains and there is sleep diary evidence that the patient has been adherent, then the clinician needs to reassess the case. Important questions at this juncture include, Is there evidence

- that the insomnia is largely "sleep state misperception?"
- that there is more physiologic arousal present in this case than is typical with primary insomnia?
- that there is circadian dysrhythmia that has not been detected or attended to ... ?
- of occult sleep disturbance or medical/psychiatric illness that not been detected or attended to ... ?
- of a substance use or abuse component that not been detected or attended to ... ?

Sleep State Misperception? (Paradixical Insomnia)

As indicated in Session 3, if the patient has a large component of sleep state misperception as part of her/his primary insomnia, this form of insomnia may not be responsive, or as responsive, to traditional CBT-I (e.g., 64). To determine whether this may be a significant factor, one can refer the patient for a PSG study or undertake an additional assessment where the patient's sleep is monitored with both actigraphy and sleep diary measures.

The issue this raises is, "Why not assess for sleep state misperception during the baseline week?" The answer is that sleep state misperception is not a contraindication for CBT-I. At this time it is unknown whether patients with substantial subjective–objective discrepancies are less responsive, or nonresponsive, to CBT-I. The assessment at this point is to explain nonresponse and to rule out the alternatives listed above as the primary moderators of nonresponse.

If it is determined that the patient does have a substantial sleep state misperception component to their insomnia, the clinician will need to (1) provide the patient some insight into this condition and (2) experiment with each of the treatment modalities to see if any, and which, yield therapeutic benefits.

With respect to providing the patient insight, the following dialogue may serve as an example of how such an issue is addressed.

Dialogue #23: Discussion of Sleep State Misperception

Therapist: The data we've collected over the last week suggests that you have a rare form of insomnia, one that we don't understand well. Let me tell you what we do know. The actigraph data we collected suggests that if we were to do a sleep study on you

- there would be no evidence of other sleep disorders that might explain your insomnia and
- the measure of your brain activity during the night, would yield something that looks like normal sleep.

Yet despite the "picture" of perfect (or near perfect) sleep, you would report in the morning that you took a long time to fall sleep and/or that you were awake for long periods of time during the night. In short, there would be a mismatch between our measure of your sleep and your sensation of it.

Patient: What do you mean? Are you saying that people would think I was lying or making this up?

Therapist: No, it's not a question of anyone thinking that your lying or making stuff up. It's just that we don't know what to make of this scenario. What's important for you to know is that there is a fair amount of research going on in this area and that there are some good ideas on the table.

One idea is that there is a kind of brain activity that is not typically measured with traditional sleep studies and that this activity is associated with a level of "engagement" or "consciousness" that normally does not occur with sleep.

- By engagement or consciousness, I mean a level of awareness during sleep that is not typical.
- By engagement or consciousness, I mean the ability to remember events that occur during sleep that most people forget.

It's not that you can do calculus during your sleep or play tapes during your sleep and learn a second language, it's just if a tape were playing, you would be more aware of this than other people. Most folks wouldn't "hear" the tape in the first place and, if they did, they wouldn't remember hearing it the next morning.

You on the other hand, while not necessarily remembering that the tape was playing or what it said, might recognize more of the information from the tape if it were played to you during the day.

But whether you recognize or remember that the tape was playing or recognize or remember "what was played," you would have the sense that it took you a long time to fall asleep and/or that you were awake for large swatches of time during the night and you would likely perceive your sleep as having been shallow.

So the question for us, is how do we change that kind of brain activity and/or derail your awareness of things going on while you're otherwise asleep.

We don't know.

What we do know, given our experience with your treatment to date, is that sleep restriction (turning up the homeostat) and stimulus control (promoting a good association between bed/bedroom/ bedtime and sleep) won't do it. Let me explain some treatment alternatives and lets make a decision about where we might go from here.

Possible candidates include relaxation training and use of sedative hypnotics. With respect to the last of these, it has been hypothesized that sleep state misperception occurs in association with increased sensory and information processing at and around sleep onset and during early NREM sleep and with the non-engagement of the mesograde amnesia which occurs with normal EEG sleep (55;56). If this hypothetical perspective is true, or in part true, it suggests that this form of insomnia is best treated with hypnotics

that are known to reduce sensory and information processing and the formation of long term memory. Thus, for this class of insomnia, standard benzodiazepines may produce more relief than other GABAergic substances like zolpidem and/or zaleplon. Whether such treatment can safely and effectively be maintained long-term remains an open question. Because our orientation is an empirical one, we believe such patients should be followed long term. Continued prescription of such controlled substances should be contingent on the patient continuing to keep sleep diaries and meeting with the therapist on a regular basis.

Physiologic Arousal?

While difficult to assay, some patients do report physiologic hyperarousal and this aspect of their insomnia may be sufficiently strong as to resist the increase in the homeostatic pressure for sleep that is produced by sleep restriction. In this scenario there are two potential solutions: (1) continue to increase sleep pressure by further delaying the patient's time to bed or (2) directly address the issue of physiologic hyperarousal by augmenting standard CBT-I with some form of relaxation training. As indicated in the early portion of this text, we're not inclined to further delay time to bed once a benchmark has been established. Given this bias, it may be useful to augment treatment with relaxation training. As noted earlier, there are at least three types of relaxation training (e.g., Diaphragmatic Breathing, Progressive Muscle Relaxation, Autogenic Training). For detailed descriptions of these methods the reader is referred to the four books that were referenced earlier in Chapter 3 of this manual.

If one of these forms of therapy is added to the clinical regimen, the clinician may elect to continue treatment for 1 to 2 additional sessions. If augmenting treatment in this way does not produce the desired outcomes, within this time frame, the clinician should consider each of the remaining alternatives.

Circadian Dysrhythmia?

The International Classification of Sleep Disorders (ICSD) nosology has a variety of disorders that fall within the broad category of Circadian Rhythm Sleep Disorders. While these are conceptualized as categorically distinct diagnostic entities, many clinical researchers feel that these kinds of disturbances exist along a continuum and may be prominent features in what is otherwise clearly primary insomnia (e.g., 65). In the context of the present discussion, nonresponse or poor response to CBT-I may suggest that circadian dysrhythmia may be a potential feature of the sleep problem that requires attention. Such patients may benefit from augmenting standard CBT-I with either phototherapy (bright light therapy) or melatonin. For additional information on this topic, the reader is referred to Lack et al.,

Circadian rhythm factors in insomnia and their treatment. In: *Treating Sleep Disorders: The Principles and Practice of Behavioral Sleep Medicine* (2003). If phototherapy is added to the clinical regimen, the clinician may elect to continue treatment for 1 to 2 more sessions.

Occult Sleep Disturbance or Medical/Psychiatric Illness?

In both instances, it is likely that the therapist will need to recommend that the patient undergo further assessment. In the case of occult sleep disorders, a PSG study would be indicated in order to answer the question "is there an intrinsic sleep disorder at play for which the patient does not show the traditional signs and symptoms?" In the case of occult medical illness, a full physical and clinical chemistries panel is now warranted. A direct discussion with the patient's primary care provider expressing concern about the lack of clinical gains and the wish to collaborate on the case is likely to be welcome.

Substance Use or Abuse?

A frank discussion with the patient about his/her substance use may or may not be productive. Reminding the patient that the pursuit of information is strictly for the purpose of explaining what factors may be interfering with treatment may precipitate, at this point, an honest exchange. If the patient is not forthcoming, the PSG may yield signs of substance use or abuse (increased REM latency, decreased total REM sleep time [alcohol abuse related artifact], increased Sigma activity in the sleep EEG [BZ or GABA receptor agonist artifact]) or direct information may be obtained from the clinical chemistries (if a comprehensive drug toxicology screen is requested).

For the last two scenarios (occult sleep disturbance or medical/psychiatric illness, substance use or abuse) it is likely that the referral for further assessment will be the end point of therapy. The patient should be informed of this and encouraged by the knowledge that you will collaborate with the referral to track down the "root of the problem." Once again, let the patient know that once the occult disorder is diagnosed and stable you will be available and will guarantee expedited access to services in the future.

Session Five: Sleep Titration (60 to 90 Minutes)

Tasks

Summarize and Graph Sleep Diary
Assess Treatment Gains
Continue Upward Titration of TST
Cognitive Therapy for Negative Sleep Beliefs

Primary Goals of This Session

1. Review data
2. Assess treatment gains
3. Make adjustments to the patient's sleep schedule
   - In the case of positive clinical gains (SE > 90%), upwardly titrate total sleep opportunity
   - In the case of no or marginal gains (SE between 85 and 90%), maintain schedule and provide rationale to the patient
   - In the case of negative gains (SE < 85%), downwardly titrate total sleep opportunity and provide rationale to the patient
4. Conduct cognitive therapy for negative sleep beliefs
5. Continue to secure the patient's commitment to the program.

Summarize and Graph Sleep Diary

As with all in-office clinical contacts, this session begins with a review of the sleep diary and the graphing of the weekly average values. Averages should be calculated and compared to previous weeks. Assess daytime complaints and functioning. Assess compliance with sleep hygiene. Titrate sleep per average SE%.

Cognitive Therapy for Negative Sleep Beliefs: A Countering Strategy for Probability Overestimates

Cognitive restructuring is a core form of therapy for CBT for depression (66) and anxiety and panic disorders (67). Some years ago we recommended that this form of therapy could be applied to the treatment of sleep-related worry (27). While there are no efficacy or effectiveness studies on this specific approach as a monotherapy, there are effectiveness data related to its use as part of a comprehensive package (49;68). Moreover, its effectiveness in the related disorders (69–71) and its clear clinical utility in the treatment

of insomnia, suggest that this is an important component to include in CBT-I.

Cognitive restructuring for insomnia focuses upon catastrophic thinking and the belief that poor sleep is *likely* to have devastating consequences. While psychoeducation may also address these kinds of issues, another ingredient of cognitive restructuring lies not in disabusing the patient of erroneous beliefs, but rather in having them discover that their estimates are not necessarily factual. When undertaking this exercise with a patient, it needs to be introduced in a considerate way, one that avoids any hint that the therapist is being pedantic, patronizing, or condescending.

There are essentially 8 steps to the process.

1. Setting the stage for cognitive restructuring
2. Calculating how long the patient has had insomnia (in days)
3. Identify and record between 3 and 10 catastrophic thoughts
4. Assess the patient's probability estimates
5. Determine the actual frequency of occurrence of the anticipated "catastrophes"
6. Discuss the mismatch between the patient's estimates and the probability of catastrophic outcome
7. Create a countering mantra to the catastrophic thoughts

The following dialog will illustrate how this form of CBT is applied. For the purpose of this example, only three catastrophic thoughts will be identified. Some patients, however, have more trouble identifying the worries they experience. To provide the clinician some targets to pursue, a more comprehensive set of examples are provided in Table 4.4.

TABLE 4.4. Common Worries and Catastrophic Thoughts

If I don't get good sleep tonight then . . .	
Worry	Associated Catastrophic Thought
I'll be irritable and short with my wife	My wife will leave or divorce me
I'll be irritable and short with my kids	My kids will hate me—never speak to me again
I want to socialize well	I lose my friends
I'll do poorly at work	I'll get fired
I'll make a mistake at work	I'll kill someone
I'll make a mistake at work	I'll get sued
I'll get fired	I will be ruined financially
I'll feel poorly	I'll get sick
I'll get sick	I'll die
I'll lose my mind	I'll go crazy—have a nervous breakdown
I won't fall asleep	I'll be awake the whole night
I'll fall sleep behind the wheel	I'll total my car
I'll have an accident	I'll wreck my car and kill myself or someone else
I'll look old and unattractive	People will turn away from me in disgust.

Dialogue #24: Setting the Stage for Cognitive Restructuring

Therapist: As you may have noticed, the work we've done to date doesn't much address the role of worry in insomnia. I know that some folks think that being a worrier is what causes insomnia—and this may be so early on, in large measure, but once the insomnia is chronic, our sense is that the disorder is maintained or continues because of the factors that we have talked about (ad nauseum). If you think back to when we talked about the Spielman or Behavioral Model—can you remember the kinds of things we identified as "perpetuating factors" for insomnia?

Patient: At this point I can practically recite them like the pledge of allegiance.

Therapist: Okay, please recite the pledge.

Patient: Extending sleep opportunity, using alcohol as a sleeping pill, staying in bed no matter what. . . .

Therapist: Right. What are the three "flavors" or three ways that folks tend to extend sleep opportunity?

Patient: Going to bed early, sleeping in, and napping during the day.

Therapist: Right. And you can see that we have made some real distance by focusing our efforts on these issues. (A good time to pull out the graphs and review them with the patient.)

But the fact is, worry is not irrelevant. It can certainly bring on a bout of insomnia, and for a chronic insomnia, it can be gas to the fire.

So today I want to spend the session focused on this issue and have you play a game with me. It's a bit of a silly game but I think when we're done, the point of the game won't be lost on you.

Patient: Okay let's play.

For an example of a data table for this exercise, see Table 4.5.

TABLE 4.5. Cognitive Restructuring—Sample Table (Number of days with Insomnia *1500*)

1	2	3	4
Event	Certainty When lying awake and unable to sleep	# of event occurrences	# of event occurences given certainty
Stay awake all night	85%	1	1200
Wreck the car	80%	2	1200
Get fired	90%	0	1300

Dialogue #25: Calculating How Long the Patient Has Had Insomnia (in Days)

Therapist: Let's start by figuring out how long you've had insomnia. As I recall you said that you've always been a poor sleeper, but that the insomnia really started in earnest with the birth of your first child. So that would be 10 years ago?

Patient: That's pretty good, but Erin's 11 years old now.

Therapist: Okay. And on average, how many bad insomnia nights would you say you have had per week.

Patient: Well its gotten worse with time so it's hard to say.

Therapist: Okay. In the beginning would it be fair to say 2 to 3 nights per week and now its up around 4 to 5 nights per week?

Patient: That sounds about right.

Therapist: Let's go with the low estimates and say 2 nights in the beginning 4 nights more recently and call it on average 3 nights per week for the 11 years.

Patient: Okay.

Therapist: So if there are 52 weeks in a year, let's call it 50 for the sake of easier math, and you have had insomnia for 11 years, let's call it 10 for the sake of easier math, then you have had insomnia for 500 weeks. And if you have had insomnia, on average 3 times per week, then you have had, conservatively speaking, insomnia on about 1500 nights.

Let me put this up on the board (write at the top of the chart "1500 nights").

The most important component to the next step is that the patient's worry be carried to its logical extreme: that the worst-case scenario be identified and framed as a possible event (e.g., fatigue → car wreck).

Dialogue #26: Identify and Record
Catastrophic Thoughts

Therapist: Settle back in your chair a bit. Maybe close your eyes and imagine you're in bed. Think back to a time before you sought out treatment. You've been lying in bed for 30 minutes, maybe more, what thoughts pop into your head?

Patient: Man, am I ever going to fall asleep?

Therapist: And when you think, "am I ever going to fall asleep," what's the real worry here, the worst-case scenario?

Patient: I'm going to be awake all night.

Therapist: Okay. That you're going to lie in bed awake all night. Let me put this up on the board (write in column 1: "Stay awake all night"). What other thoughts pop into your head?

Patient: If I'm up all night, I'm going to feel incredibly bad tomorrow.

Therapist: Okay. Let's say you are up all night, and you'll feel incredibly bad tomorrow. What might happen if this were to be the case?

Patient: I might wreck the car on the way to work because I am so sleep deprived.

Therapist: Is this a thought that occurs to you while your lying awake at night?

Patient: Absolutely. I think I'm going to be so fatigued and exhausted that I'm just going to run off the road and crash into a tree or something.

Therapist: Okay. Let me put this up on the board (write in column 1: "wreck the car"). What other thoughts pop into your head when you're lying in bed and thinking you're never going to fall asleep?

Patient: I'm going to be so messed up on the following day, that I'll do poorly at work.

Therapist: And when you think "I'll do poorly at work," what's the real worry here, the worst-case scenario?

Patient: I'll get fired. I lose my job.

Therapist: Okay. Let me put this up on the board (write in column 1: "get fired").

Dialogue #27: Assess the Patient's Probability Estimates

Therapist: We now have three things on the board. The question I'd like you to answer for me is this: When you're lying there in bed, wide-awake, how certain are you when you think each of these things that they are going to happen? How certain are you, at that moment when you're lying awake in bed, that you're going to "stay awake all night?"

Patient: Pretty certain.

Therapist: 100% certain? 90% certain? How convinced at that moment, when you think the thought, are you?

Patient: I don't know—maybe 85% sure.

Therapist: Okay. (Write in column 2: "85%").

How certain are you, when you're lying awake in bed awake, that you're going to "wreck the car?"

Patient: Maybe 80% sure. It's hard to say, because I feel differently about things under those circumstances.

Therapist: I know. Hold that thought. (Write in column 2: "80%").
    One more to go. How certain are you, when you're lying awake in bed awake, that you're going to "get fired?"

Patient: 90% sure. I worry about this a lot.

Therapist: Okay. (Write in column 2: "90%").

Dialogue #28: Determine the Actual Frequency of the Anticipated Catastrophes

Therapist: Okay, on to the next column and questions.
    How many times have you gone without sleep for a whole night? On how many occasions was the insomnia so bad that you didn't sleep a wink?

Patient: That's hard to answer. Hard to know when you get one or two "winks" of sleep, but if I have to give a hard answer, maybe once—probably not even that.

Therapist: I know it's hard to tell. Let's say once for argument's sake. (Write in column 3: "once"). How many times have you slept so poorly that the next day you got into an accident—you "wrecked your car?"

Patient: Actually I have wrecked my car twice over the last 11 years, and I am certain that one of those times was insomnia related. I remember it pretty clearly.

Therapist: Okay. Let's say, for argument's sake, that both accidents were related to your insomnia (Write in column 3: "twice"). How many times have you slept so poorly that the next day you did so bad at work that your got fired?

Patient: Never. This is more a worrywart thing. I tend to rise to the occasion when it comes to work.

Therapist: Okay. (Write in column 3: "None").

Dialogue #29: Mismatch Between the Patient's Estimates and the Probability of Catastrophic Outcomes

Therapist: Here comes the game aspect to this exercise. One way of thinking about and judging the reasonableness of one's certainties is to see how well they match "the facts."

To do this we need to compare the actual occurrences of the events we've listed here with how often they should have happened given your level of certainty and the number of opportunities you have had for the events to have occurred.

Let's start with *staying awake all night.* If you've had insomnia for 1500 nights and your certainty about the possibility of staying awake all night were reasonable, you'd have experienced it on 85% of the occasions when you had a bout of insomnia, so that would be .85 × 1500, or 1275 times. Hmmm—Let's call it 1200 times. (Write in column 4: "1200").

Lets take the example of *wrecking your car.* If you've had insomnia for 1500 nights and your certainty about the possibility of wrecking your car were reasonable, you'd have experienced it on 80% of the occasions when you had a bout of insomnia, so that would be .80 × 1500, or 1200 times. (Write in column 4: "1200").

Lets take the example of *getting fired.* If you've had insomnia for 1500 nights and your certainty about the possibility of getting fired were reasonable, you'd have experienced it on 90% of the occasions when you had a bout of insomnia, so that would be .90 × 1500, or 1350 times. Let's call it 1300 times. (Write in column 4: "1300").

So here's the interesting bit. Somehow when your lying in bed it seems reasonable to think, and to be very certain of the accuracy of it, that its likely

- that you'll stay awake all night,
- that you'll wreck the car,
- that you'll get fired,

but your experience tells you otherwise. Your experience tells you that these are actually "low probability events." In fact unbelievably low probability events. Given the number of occurrences to date, the probabilities are closer to

0.06%	incidence of not falling asleep	(versus 85%)
0.13%	incidence of wrecking the car	(versus 80%)
0%	incidence of getting fired	(versus 90%)

In other words, all these events, which seem like such imminent possibilities when you're trying to fall asleep, actually have less than a 1% probability of actually occurring.

Dialogue #30: Create a Countering Mantra to the Catastrophic Thoughts

Therapist: *Bottom line:* When you are having trouble falling asleep and you start thinking the "If I don't fall asleep I may," it helps to counter with "I may not. . . . In fact, it's downright unlikely that I may. . . ." Just thinking "not likely" when you have catastrophic worries is helpful. We like to refer to this as a countering "mantra." A thing that you can say in your head and it sort of promotes "relaxation"—"de-stressing."
    Try it—think "not likely." Let's take an example.

Patient: I'll be so fatigued tomorrow that I'll wreck my car.

Therapist: How likely is this given how may times you've driven to work after a bad nights sleep?

Patient: Not very.

Therapist: Now that's the ticket!

Session Six: Sleep Titration (30 to 60 Minutes)

Tasks

Summarize and Graph Sleep Diary
Assess Treatment Gains
Follow Up: Negative Sleep Beliefs
Continue Upward Titration of TST

Primary Goals of This Session

1. Review data
2. Assess treatment gains
3. Make adjustments to the patient's sleep schedule
   - In the case of positive clinical gains (SE > 90%), upwardly titrate total sleep opportunity
   - In the case of no or marginal gains (SE between 85 and 90%), maintain schedule and provide rationale to the patient
   - In the case of negative gains (SE < 85%), downwardly titrate total sleep opportunity and provide rationale to the patient
4. Address remaining issues regarding intrusive thoughts and negative sleep beliefs
5. Continue to secure the patient's commitment to the program

Summarize and Graph Sleep Diary

As with all in-office clinical contacts, this session begins with a review of the sleep diary and the graphing of the weekly average values. Averages should be calculated and compared to previous weeks. Assess daytime complaints and functioning. Assess complaints with sleep hygiene. Titrate sleep per average SE.

NOTE: Some clinicians use a 6-session model and thus cover relapse prevention strategies in this session. In the present model the sixth and seventh sessions are primarily to make sure that the patient is maintaining his/her "forward momentum." These sessions may also be used to provide adjunctive/adjuvant treatment (relaxation training, bright light therapy, additional cognitive therapy, and so on) for patients that exhibit only partial response. Currently, there is no formal definition for what constitutes a "partial response." A good rule of thumb is to monitor the patient's own sense of accomplishment. How satisfied are they with treatment? Do they feel that they "should" make more progress than they have?

Session Seven: Sleep Titration (30 to 60 Minutes)

> ## *Tasks*
>
> Summarize and Graph Sleep Diary
> Assess Treatment Gains
> Follow Up: Negative Sleep Beliefs
> Continue Upward Titration of TST

Primary Goals of This Session

1. Review data
2. Assess treatment gains
3. Make adjustments to the patient's sleep schedule
   - In the case of positive clinical gains (SE > 90%), upwardly titrate total sleep opportunity
   - In the case of no or marginal gains (SE between 85 and 90%), maintain schedule and provide rationale to the patient
   - In the case of negative gains (SE < 85%), downwardly titrate total sleep opportunity and provide rationale to the patient
4. Address remaining issues regarding intrusive thoughts and negative sleep beliefs
5. Continue to secure the patient's commitment to the program

Summarize and Graph Sleep Diary

As with all in-office clinical contacts, this session begins with a review of the sleep diary and the graphing of the weekly average values. Averages should be calculated and compared to previous weeks. Assess daytime complaints and functioning. Assess complaints with sleep hygiene. Titrate sleep per average SE.

As with the previous session, this session may also be used to provide adjunctive/adjuvant treatment (relaxation training, bright light therapy, additional cognitive therapy, and so on) for patients that exhibit only partial response.

Session Eight: Sleep Titration (30 to 60 Minutes)

Tasks

Summarize and Graph Sleep Diary
Assess Treatment Gains (Globally)
Discuss Relapse Prevention

Primary Goals of This Session

1. Review data (weekly values)
2. Assess treatment gains
3. Discuss Relapse Prevention
   - review behavioral perspective on insomnia
   - discuss the approach to maintaining clinical gains
   - discuss what to do when the insomnia returns

Summarize and Graph Sleep Diary (Weekly Values)

As with all in-office clinical contacts, this session begins with a review of the sleep diary and the graphing of the weekly average values.

Assess Treatment Gains

Extra time should be taken in this session to review treatment gains for the whole of the treatment interval, with a particular emphasis on the patient's gains from the baseline. This can be accomplished by framing the data in terms of pre-post change for all the sleep continuity parameters and/or by illustrating the change with treatment using the chart progress graphs. Be sure to emphasize that the longitudinal data suggest that treatment gains are extremely durable with time (72;73).

Discuss Relapse Prevention

Review Behavioral Perspective on Insomnia

Reviews "how insomnia gets started" (referring again to the Spielman/ Behavioral Model) and how it gets maintained over time. One way to accomplish this task would be to *have the patient draw the model* on the dry erase board and then explain to the therapist what the predisposing, precipitating, and perpetuating factors are, and to provide specific examples that apply to their situation. This kind of exchange might also provide an

opportunity for the patient and the clinician to identify risk factors for occurrence and what steps might be taken to reduce their risk.

Discuss the Approach to Maintaining Clinical Gains

The main issue here is, when discontinuing supervised treatment, what aspects of treatment need and don't need to be carried forward. Assuming that treatment has gone well, there are a variety of things that the patient will not need to do anymore, or at least not on a regular basis. For example, with time it may be permissible to engage in behaviors in the bedroom other than sex and sleep (e.g., reading in bed). There are, however, a variety of prescriptions that should be continued or only gradually phased out. An example of a prescription that is likely to be long term is the provision that bedtime and waketime be stable—if not fixed. Whether one carries forward the sleep schedule as fixed or flexible is judged on a case-by-case basis. Some patients, such as those who suffer from idiopathic (life-long) insomnia, may be best served by maintaining a strict schedule that does not vary with time. Other patients, perhaps the majority, may do better by allowing for a slow, continued upward titration of TIB/TST. For these individuals, once upward titration is discontinued and regular bedtimes and wake times are established, it may be possible for the patient to consider these scheduled times as guideposts. That is, deviating from the schedule need not represent relapse. One night of a rigid schedule did not fix their sleep and one "night off" is unlikely to break it. Therefore it may be possible that on one or two nights a week the patient may not set an alarm and sleep in a bit longer. This can only work if the patient returns to their regular schedule for the majority of the week. This schedule might feel more normal. If this is pursued, it should only be done provided that several caveats are borne in mind. First, the patient should only sleep in on predetermined days, for example, weekends, and never sleep in following a bad night. Extending sleep opportunity following a poor night's sleep would be compensatory and may result in an acute bout of insomnia. The amount of extra sleep allowed on the "flex days" should be restricted to no more than 30 to 60 minutes as longer intervals risk depriming the homeostat. Second, when sleeping in the patient may find that, despite not setting an alarm, she/he might wake at her/his usual time. In such instances the patient should allow herself/himself the opportunity to go back to sleep provided that only a brief amount of time is spent awake in bed. Here again stimulus control rules are useful such that one should only stay awake in bed for a short time interval (i.e., 15 minutes or less) and he/she should leave the bedroom when having the sensation that he/she are "wide awake" or experiencing irritation about not being able to return to sleep.

Augmenting Clinical Gains

It may be argued that when CBT-I is practiced in the standardized fashion (as is described throughout this manual) that the termination of treatment at the close of 6 to 8 sessions is premature. If this is the case, then it should be true that there is more that the patient can do, outside of proper therapy, to augment their clinical gains.

The evidence for the notion that treatment has been terminated prematurely is that there is little to no pre/post change in TST. That is, by the end of therapy, TST usually only reaches a level that is comparable to, or slightly exceeds, baseline measures. In fact, the average increase in TST over baseline is about 6% (4).

One line of thought regarding the minimal TST gains is that this is not actually evidence that more therapy is needed or that there is more that the patient can do to "get better." Instead, TST is conceived of as a proxy variable for sleep need. Sleep need, in turn, is considered to be a stable "trait" characteristic. Thus, the goal of therapy is not to increase sleep need, but only to make sure that sleep is easy to initiate and reinitiate and that one sleeps efficiently. Accordingly, there is nothing for the patient to do to augment their clinical gains.

The other line of thought, which is frankly more in line with the longitudinal studies of insomnia, is that TST may increase with time and without the need for further intervention. These improvements can be ascribed to a variety of considerations including: the long-term effects of good stimulus control over sleep, deconditioning of arousal, change in the negative beliefs about sleep and sleep loss, the persistent effects of good sleep hygiene, and so on. Thus, while the patient may expect to improve with time, (see Figure 4.2); there is nothing for the patient to do to augment clinical gains beyond engaging in good maintenance practices and careful management of acute recurrences.

Discuss What to Do When Insomnia Recurs

The primary idea to instill is the notion that the patient will again experience insomnia and that transient bouts are to be expected and are normal. There is even the possibility that acute insomnia has some value toward dealing with transient life stress. The patient needs to be reminded that lots of things may trigger a bout of insomnia and the main thing one can do to protect against a new onset episode of *chronic insomnia* is: (1) to not compensate for sleep loss, (2) to engage stimulus control procedures immediately, and (3) to reengage sleep restriction should the insomnia persist beyond a few days. If the insomnia continues (persisting for 1–2 weeks), the patient should know that they are always welcome to come back into treatment and they will be guaranteed expedited access to what will probably be short-term treatment. Below is an example of an exchange between the clinician and patient regarding the topic of recurrence.

Dialogue #31: What Happens If I Stop Sleeping Again?

Patient: So what happens if I have problems sleeping again?

Therapist: Well, what do you think the first thing to do is when you have a bad night?

Patient: Restrict?

Therapist: Well, that may be jumping the gun. Sleep restriction is really a procedure aimed at dealing with insomnia when it is chronic where homeostatic pressure is used to promote short sleep latency and increased sleep efficiency. At this point, that is not your problem. You just happen to be awake, and what we want to do is to not pair being awake again with bedtime, bedroom, and so on. To deal with that problem, what do you think you should do?

Patient: Not be in bed!

Therapist: Bingo. This aspect of stimulus control is forever. There is no good purpose served by remaining in bed for protracted periods of time upset and/or awake. Remember the rule, the moment you know you are awake, and/or annoyed about it, you are out of bed.

But, let's say the worst happens, you activate stimulus control, and the insomnia continues over several days (say a week), then what should you do?

Patient: Restrict?

Therapist: Yep. So what does that mean?

Patient: So, I'm supposed to keep a diary like for a week, then at the end of the week, calculate the averages for total sleep time and time in bed and then use these to setup a new sleep schedule. That is, I will subtract my total sleep time from the time I need to get up in the morning, and that will be my bedtime for the next week.

Therapist: Sounds right, give me an example.

Patient: Suppose that I calculate that I am averaging 5 hours of sleep for the last week, and I need to get up at 6 AM. That means that I should set my bedtime for 1 AM.

Therapist: "Right you are." What is the next step?

Patient: I get 15 minutes back every week if my sleep efficiency is >90%, I stay the same if it is between 85% and 90%, and I restrict even further if it is <85%. So how long am I supposed to do this?

Therapist: That is a good question. If you are being successful on your own, and you reestablish reasonable sleep times and sleep efficiency, that's great. On the other hand if you find it is difficult for you to do this my yourself, or you are concerned that there are new factors at play that may require new evaluation, then you know where to find me. One thing that I can guarantee you, is that you will get expedited access to service.

Finally, it is worth noting that treatment gains are most often maintained or improved over time. That is, relapse rates are small provided all things remain equal, (no new illness, childbirths, etc) and the patient continues good habits. Of the patients that experience relapses, the story seems invariably the same. That is, the patient has done well for quite some time, but at some point started having transient bouts of insomnia which they ignored up to that point as they had been sleeping well. However, after some time passes, panic may set in and instead of engaging in self guided SCT and SRT, patients tend to engage in the same behaviors that perpetuated the index episode. If this pattern continues, the patient will have waited too long and is likely to experience another bout of chronic insomnia. When treat-

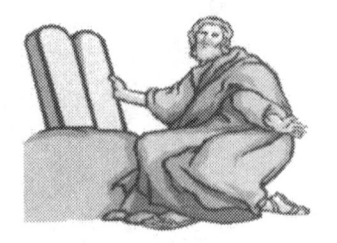

Two commandments to keep holy:

I. never stay in bed awake 10-15 minutes (or upset, frustrated, or even just alert).
II. never compensate for a bad night.

don't turn in early, stay in bed later, or nap

Remember The Mantra:

If not tonight – then tomorrow night.

That is – I may sleep poorly tonight but tomorrow night
I'm increasingly likely to sleep well.

FIGURE 4.3. Two Commandments of Relapse Prevention.

ment is reinitiated, these patients tend to exhibit an accelerated recovery. Interestingly, such patients while clear on the procedures to be engaged in, do better in a brief therapy context where they are coached through the first few sessions. In the final analysis, the take home message is, "don't let the small burning embers of transient insomnia accelerate into a blaze."

The session ends by providing the patient a handout to help remind them how to maintain their gains (see Figure 4.3).

5
CBT-I Example Dialogues for Patient Questions and Challenges

The following pages focus on the concerns or problems that patients encounter while in Cognitive Behavioral Therapy for Insomnia (CBT-I). Many, if not all, of these areas of concern run throughout the entire course of therapy rather than being specifically related to one session or another. Accordingly, in this section of the manual, we will organize the discussion by content area, as opposed to by session number.

Concerns About the Sleep Diaries

Sleep diaries are central to the conduct of CBT-I. They are the data source for this data-driven form of therapy. Interestingly, as important as they are for treatment, some patients have difficulty complying with this pivotal aspect of therapy. For some patients, the concern will be related to whether or not they can accurately report the data (especially given the initial recommendation to not watch the clock). For other patients, the task itself may be too alien or may seem redundant with the information they provided during the intake interview. For yet other patients, the issue may be related to the lack of objective measurement.

Questions Related to Accuracy of Reporting

Dialogue #32: I'm Having Trouble Filling Out the Sleep Diaries

Patient: If I'm not to watch the clock, how will I know what to write on my diary?

Therapist: Most people have a pretty good sense of how much time has elapsed and can make reasonable estimates regarding such things

as "how long did it take you to fall sleep," "how much time did you spend awake after you first fell asleep," and so on. When we measure these things using fancy equipment, we'd find that most people estimate these variables pretty accurately, say between 5 and 30 minutes of what the objective measures show.

It's true that some people are more inaccurate about these judgments, but even in these cases these folks are inaccurate in a reasonably reliable way—and this is the most important thing for us. If all your estimates are reliably off, we are still able to monitor how these estimates change with treatment—and at the end of the day—it's the change (the measurement of improvement) that we're interested in.

Patient: What if I can't tell if I'm awake or I'm asleep?

Therapist: Do the best you can. For our purposes there are no in-between categories. You're either awake or asleep. Just pick what you think it is and write it on the diary. The only incorrect diary entries are "no entries" or question marks, etc. Always put down a number. We'll assume that the number represents your best guess.

If you'd like a rule of thumb, I can offer this: if you're not sure, it is likely that for a lot of the time in question, you were awake, so just count it as "wake."

Patient: Sometimes it feels like I wake up lots of times from very short periods of sleep. What should I do about that?

Therapist: As always, depends on what the question is. If the question is "How many times did you awaken last night, after initially falling asleep?" Then make your best guess.

For example, if you feel like you woke up a dozen times, the number you should record is "12." If you feel like you were awake only a minute or two, then when asked "how much time were you awake after you initially fell asleep," then pick the number between 12 and 24 minutes that feels right to you, the one that best represents your sensation of how much time you were awake.

Patient: What about naps? I almost never nap, but sometimes I lie down and rest, although I never actually sleep. How am I supposed to record this?

Therapist: Over the course of therapy, we'll talk a lot about the issue of "knowing when you're asleep" or the "perception of sleep." For the time being, when you record napping on the sleep diaries just assume you slept the whole time, unless your certain about how much you did or didn't sleep during the nap.

Questions Related to the Need to Complete Daily Diaries

Dialogue #33: Why Do I Have to Fill Out Sleep Diaries?

Patient: I don't understand. I completed all the sleep questionnaires and now I have to do this with the diaries as well. Why isn't the information I already provided adequate?

Therapist: Good question. Lots of the information you provided on the questionnaires is just fine, and there is no need for us to gather additional data. But in the case specifically related to your sleep complaint, we need to gather information on a daily basis for a week or two, so that we can see how much variability there is from day to day and what factors might contribute to this.

Beyond this there is the whole issue of how folks come to form impressions regarding their illness and, for that matter, how people come to form impressions about anything that occurs in their lives on a variable basis. Most of us don't remember every instance (and maybe this is a good thing). Most people come up with "rules of thumb." The big three rules of thumb that most of us use to form generalizations are: primacy, saliency, and recency. These are useful heuristics (ways of coming up with generalizations), but unfortunately they tend to bias people's "averages" towards extremes. The diaries allow us to get around this and to base our averages on the repeated measure of the things we're interested in.

Questions Related to the Lack of Objective Measurement

Dialogue #34: Shouldn't We Use Fancy Equipment to Measure My Sleep?

Patient: I am really surprised that there is no flashy equipment to measure my sleep and that you rely on "diaries." Even the term is a little unsettling. I feel like I should be keeping notes on my love life.

Therapist: I hear you. Rest assured we will not ask you to gather any data on your love life.

As you can see from the format of the diaries, we're interested in very specific things, most of which are just related to your day-to-day impressions of your sleep. The term "diary" may be an unfortunate

one because it doesn't give credence to the value of repeated measure assessment. The data we gather in this manner are critical for our getting an accurate picture of your sleep problem and they will serve to guide your treatment.

Patient: Fine. But why self-report? Isn't there some fancy equipment you can use to gather day-to-day information on my sleep?

Therapist: As a matter fact there is. We could study your sleep in the sleep lab, or even send you home with some ambulatory monitoring equipment. And we may yet do this. But our experience is that in most cases, the day-to-day self-report data provides what we need to effectively diagnose and treat your insomnia.

Patient: If you say so, but how can this be better than an objective measure?

Therapist: There's that word again: "Better." It's true that the fancy equipment is more objective and it's also true that such equipment allows us to look at factors that we cannot assess with sleep diaries. But for now, the factor we're most interested in is the one that brought you in for treatment in the first place; the fact that you *feel* that you are not sleeping well.

What's critical for us is that we programmatically and systematically change your feeling that you don't sleep well. If we're not successful in doing this within the next 2 to 4 weeks, then we get out the fancy equipment to look for what might have been missed. Make sense?

Patient: Yes. But why not save the step and do the fancy evaluation upfront?

Therapist: Truth. The "fancy" procedures are expensive and neither you nor your insurance company will want to pay for such things unless they're truly indicated. In this case, indicated means that you require further evaluation because you did not respond to first line treatment. But lest I be too cynical, the vast majority of patients that are seen in this service improve and maintain their gains without ever needing additional evaluation. So there is some wisdom in waiting for the fancy stuff to be indicated before conducting such procedures.

Questions Related to the Ability to Complete the Daily Diaries

---

Dialogue #35: I Can't Seem to Remember to Fill Out My Diary

Patient: I can't seem to remember to fill out my diary each day. Sometimes later in the day I will remember, but then it's hard to get the numbers straight. So I decide to just try to do better tomorrow, but I always seem to forget.

Therapist: As you know, we really need these data. So let's figure out a way that will help you to remember.

One thing you can try is to put the diary on your pillow each morning so that when you return to bed at night it will be there to remind you to fill it out. Then put the diary on the floor approximately where your feet will land when you get out of bed in the morning. Again that will force you to see the diary, at which point you can remember to fill it out quickly and to place it back on your pillow.

Medication Issues

If the patient's sleep is "perfect" on hypnotics and the patient does not want to discontinue pharmacotherapy, it is unlikely that they will be presenting for treatment. In the instances where such patients do seek treatment, their goal is usually to discontinue medication after CBT-I. Thus, the question is, "Is this a viable strategy?" We believe it is usually best to taper the client off medication before treatment begins for at least three reasons. First, it will allow for the clinician to establish a baseline for what the patient's sleep looks like when he/she is medication free. Second, it helps avoid posttreatment withdrawal. That is, the patient may make substantial gains with CBT-I only to have those gains temporarily reversed when medication is discontinued during or following therapy. Third, concomitant use of hypnotics along with CBT-I may interfere with the patient's attributions regarding the efficacy of CBT-I.

It should be noted, however, that it is often the case that the patient's sleep is not "perfect" on hypnotics, especially if medication has been used for an extended period of time. Several studies show that the sleep of patients with insomnia on and off medication is remarkably similar (74). A final testament to this is that many patients seek CBT-I treatment while they continue to use sedatives. This probably occurs, in part, because the patient does not wish to continuously take medications, and in part, because medications have not provided whatever constitutes "good sleep." Thus it

is likely that the majority of patients will be interested in, and compliant with, the effort to discontinue pharmacotherapy—and to do so at treatment initiation.

Finally, there is this question, "Do hypnotics have sustained efficacy and or a curative potential?" In the absence of data to suggest otherwise, it would appear that the long-term use of sedative hypnotics is palliative. At best, medications provide good symptom relief, so long as the patient is maintained on the medication. At worst, some or all of the sedative hypnotics produce tolerance, promote rebound insomnia, and suppress the forms of sleep that are thought to have functions such as memory consolidation (75–78), mood regulation (79–81), and tissue restoration (82;83). This is especially true of benzodiazepines and is less likely to apply to the new generation sedatives of the non-benzo benzodiazepine class. Given the worst-case scenario, and the demonstrated long-term efficacy of CBT-I, the most rational course of treatment is to have the patient discontinue the use of hypnotics. The following dialogue serves to illustrate how the subject of medication discontinuation is broached with the patient.

Dialogue #36: I'm Really Nervous About Stopping My Sleeping Pills

Patient: If I'm going to get off of my sleep meds, can I wait until we are done with the treatment?

Therapist: The goal is to have you stop taking medication *before* treatment starts. There are several reasons for this, not the least of which is we need to have a clear understanding of what your sleep looks like when you're not using the sleep meds.

Patient: I can tell you what that's like because I stopped it three weeks ago for one night, and I didn't sleep at all.

Therapist: I can well imagine. These medications when stopped abruptly can cause what we refer to as "rebound insomnia." This means a recurrence of your insomnia in a form that is probably more severe than what you had before starting medication. This is a drug effect and not a matter of unmasking your insomnia, as it exists today. It is probably also the case that there are psychological factors at play. That is, you may have believed that you wouldn't sleep without the sleep meds and when you stopped taking them you probably started worrying about your sleep. The combination of your expectation and worry probably compounded the problem that occurred simply because of the withdrawal. The result: "you didn't sleep at all."

Patient: So what can I do? I can't go through that again, it was pure torture.

Therapist: The plan is to wean you more slowly off the medication to minimize the withdrawal. Although you will sleep worse for a short time, once you are completely off for a week or so, you may find that your sleep spontaneously gets better. For many of our patients who use hypnotics chronically, once past the withdrawal they find that their sleep is as good as it was before using medications. And in many patients, they find (ironically) that once past the withdrawal, their sleep is about the same on or off medication.

Patient: Hmm, that is interesting. What is the other reason to stop the medication now?

Therapist: Right. The treatment requires some hard work on your part and will take time to return you to good sleep. We don't want you to go through all that work, start to sleep well, and *then* wean off medication. This will only result in the withdrawal we just spoke about and cause your sleep to deteriorate again for a while.

Patient: So, you're saying it's better to just get it over with and then fix my sleep.

Therapist: Exactly!

Patient: What if my doctor does not want me to stop using my medication?

Therapist: In most cases, physicians are more than happy to have you decrease your use of sleep medications. This is so because there is a clear consensus that hypnotics do not "cure," do not produce normal sleep, and they may be psychologically addictive. So, in all likelihood it will be fine with your doctor. But, to make sure we are all on the same page and that we are approaching your care in a collaborative way, I will (with your permission) speak with your doctor and together we will develop a plan.

Patient: Well actually I think it will be fine, so I'll just get off the medication starting tonight.

Therapist: As we've talked about before, we need to consult with your physician and put together a plan for weaning you off of the medication. We want to maximize the likelihood of a smooth and successful taper.

Patient: What's the big deal? Six months ago I wasn't taking these medications so why not just go back to that now? It can't hurt me!

Therapist: You're right. It's not *likely* to hurt you. But it is *possible.* Sometimes a quick withdrawal can not only be uncomfortable, but dangerous. As we spoke about earlier, coming off too quickly can cause seizures, depending on the medication. So it's really best that we consult with your physician and work with him/her collaboratively.

How to Approach a Patient Who Hasn't Carried Out the Taper?

Dialogue #37: I Tried But Couldn't Stop Taking My Sleeping Pills

Therapist: I see from your diaries that you still are taking sleeping pills. What happened to the taper?

Patient: Well I tried to get off the medication, but after three days of not sleeping I couldn't take it anymore so I went back on it.

Therapist: There is no doubt that this is hard. Sad to say this will almost certainly take longer than three days. It may take a week or more for your system to return to normal. As with everything, consistency is the key. When you stopped for three days and then went back on the medication, you essentially suffered for no reason. So, it would be better not to start this process again until you are ready to see it through. Once you start reducing medication, the goal is to get off and stay off until the end no matter what. Maybe it will help to think of it this way: this will be a lot easier than say quitting smoking or drinking. One week and its done.

Patient: Will I ever go back on medication?

Therapist: Our hope, if you are successful in this therapy, is that you won't ever need to use sleeping pills on a regular basis again.

Patient: I don't know if I can do this. I think I will get three days in and give in again.

Therapist: You may want to keep in mind that there is a light at the end of the tunnel and you have to stay the course to get there. If you keep going halfway into the tunnel and then turn around and come out, you are just not going to get where you are going, and you will be in the position of needing to start all over again. The moral of the story: once in the tunnel, follow the light and don't stop until you are on the other side.

Patient: What if I never get there?

Therapist: It is our sincere belief that if you do the work correctly, you will get to the other side. Should we find, however, that after a week or two that this is not working for you—no matter what adjustments we make—we can then always go back to using medications.

Possibly different medications than you are using now. But we will cross that bridge when we come to it. For now the job is to forge ahead in the tunnel.

Patient: What happens if the sleep loss goes on for longer than a few days . . . what happens if the sleep loss goes on for a few weeks. Can't it hurt me not to sleep at all?

Therapist: Yes. But the amount of sleep loss has to be pretty substantial. If we extrapolate from animal data we'd be talking months of *total sleep deprivation* to produce serious illness and even here this would be reversible. The main thing to remember is there is a trade off. It's like what athletes say "no pain, no gain."

Concerns About the Negative Effects of Treatment

How does one approach a person who is worried that the transient negative side effects of CBT-I will interfere with their daily function? Please note that this issue is also covered in Session Two, with the dialogue that discusses the relationship between short and long term gain (see also Figure 4.2).

Dialogue #38: If I Don't Get to Sleep, How Am I Going to Function?

Patient: Okay. Fine. I'm not going to die or get supersick. But what about the effect of my not sleeping or sleeping well on my work? I have an important job, and I have to be at my best. I can't afford to be sleep deprived!

Therapist: I understand. What happened in the past, before you were using medication?

Patient: Oh it was awful! I was sluggish, drowsy, and I couldn't think straight. I just couldn't function!

Therapist: So you stopped going to work?

Patient: No, I went to work, but it was miserable.

Therapist: And while you were there, did you get any work done at all?

Patient: Well some, but not as much as I would have liked.

Therapist: Did anybody at work comment on that?

Patient: Lots of people said I looked tired.

Therapist: Yes, but did they comment on your work?

Patient: No, not exactly.

Therapist: Did you make any big mistakes that came back to haunt you or put your job in jeopardy?

Patient: No nothing like that.

Therapist: How long were you having trouble sleeping before you went on medications?

Patient: At least four months.

Therapist: So during that time you were sleep deprived, but you functioned well enough at work to get things done and not get fired!

Patient: Yes, but it was hard!

Therapist: Of course. I am certain that it was very hard, but you didn't really stop functioning at all. You felt tired and lousy but functioned reasonably well. And you didn't come down with a terrible illness either.

Patient: I can't just live like that!

Therapist: And nobody is asking you to. Remember, the plan is to keep you off medications long enough to clear your system. Then, we will work together in an efficient manner to get your sleep back on track. Like when the insomnia started, you're facing several weeks of poor sleep and feeling poorly. Unlike when the insomnia started, this time you have a goal to shoot for and a plan. This time there's "a light at the end of the tunnel."

How does one approach a person who is worried that the transient negative side effects of CBT-I will interfere with their daily function and who has experienced negative outcomes that are related to, or attributed to, poor sleep?

The "trick" here is to find some aspect of the patient's life that worked during the period of time when he/she experienced negative outcomes. The idea is to get him/her to focus on the fact that it was his/her discomfort that was disabling and not an inability to function on his/her part. Once he/she understands this, he/she may be more willing to tolerate discomfort.

Dialogue #39: No, Really, There Have Been Times When I Haven't Functioned

Patient: When I was sleep deprived, I often stop seeing friends and didn't go out. It was just awful.

Therapist: Were there times when you've forced yourself to go out and see friends or go to work?

Patient: Yes, at times I had to, but it was extremely hard.

Therapist: What happened?

Patient: I would go out, but it was no fun at all. I would drag and have to push myself the entire time.

Therapist: Were you able to converse, eat meals, and so on?

Patient: Yes but. . . .

Therapist: Can you think of any specific time like this?

Patient: Yes, my grandson's graduation.

Therapist: Did you have any fun at all? Did you laugh a bit? Were you proud?

Patient: Absolutely I was proud!

Therapist: So not all of your time was completely lousy. I'm sure it was hard and you were tired, but you had some fun. Compare that to when you sat home. Did you have fun then?

Patient: No, most of the time I was fighting just to stay awake.

Therapist: Hmmm. So, on balance, not compensating had a better outcome? That is, going out and doing something (even while you didn't feel at your best) is better than letting the insomnia get the better of you (by forcing you to do something less desirable).

Patient: Yes, I guess I can see that.

Therapist: Let's take this a step further. Following a bad night, or series of bad nights, when you rearrange your life to accommodate the fact that you feel poorly, this means the insomnia necessarily had a bad outcome. That and there is no way for you to know what might have happened if you had toughed it out. Maybe things would have been okay, or better than okay. But instead, by rearranging your schedule, the only thing to be learned or experienced is that the insomnia does lead to negative things.

And if this isn't enough of a "Catch-22," accommodating the insomnia by being less active makes it more likely that the insomnia will persist, if not worsen. This is so because when you're home "compensating for sleep loss" its likely that you will be less physically active, more inclined to nap, and more likely to go to bed earlier and spend time awake in bed. All tolled, such things are almost certain to make the insomnia worse, and all in the name of trying to feel better.

How does one approach a patient who is not naïve to a part or all of the treatment protocol: "Been there, done that!"

There are two issues here. One is that the patient says, "been there, done that" and is indeed familiar with the buzzwords, but has not practiced something even remotely like the standard treatments. The classic sitcom example of this occurred on a TV show called *Doogie Howser, MD* (an episode on which Richard Bootzin actually collaborated). In this episode, Howser's friend, Vinnie Delpino, is having trouble with insomnia. He is evaluated at a sleep clinic and told to engage in stimulus control therapy (called the "Bootzin Method" on the TV show). Delpino interprets the instructions to mean that he should ride his bicycle around his bed until tired, and then return to bed. This is an interesting application of the "Bootzin Method," but one that substantially deviates from the standard form of the treatment. The point here being that when the patient says "been there, done that," what they have done may not remotely resemble what is needed.

Thus, it is imperative that the therapist begin by asking what interventions have been engaged and that the patient provide the name and details of the practice and describe the extent to which the practice was and wasn't effective. In the instance where the practice bears no resemblance to "reality," one explains to the patient the actual therapy and the important ways that it differs from what was practiced. In the instance where the practice was "standard," the therapist focuses on the fact that practice is only, or most, effective when part of a program of treatment. Below is an example dialogue.

Dialogue #40: I've Already Tried Behavioral Stuff and It Doesn't Work

Patient: I'm not sure why I am here. My physician has already worked with me on the behavioral stuff.

Therapist: You mean your primary care doctor? The person who you see for your annual physicals and when you don't feel well?

Patient: Yes.

Therapist: When you say "behavioral stuff," what do you mean?

Patient: He handed me a list of rules and then we did something called "stimulus control."

Therapist: The list, was it a list of "Do's and Don'ts" where, for example, you were told to avoid caffeinated products?

Patient: Yes. That's it.

Therapist: Right. This is referred to as sleep hygiene instructions. The idea being that there is a variety things one can do and not do that will make it easier to fall asleep and stay asleep. The idea of a good sleep "to-do list" is a good one, but too simple and too absolute. More importantly, the data clearly show that sleep hygiene instructions are not, in and of themselves, effective.

Patient: My doctor also did sleep restriction with me.

Therapist: What did this entail?

Patient: Going to bed later. He said midnight but usually I went to bed at 11:45, and got out of bed at a fixed time.

Therapist: What time did you get out of bed?

Patient: Same time as usual: 7:30 AM.

Therapist: Hmmm. Well there is certainly some similarity here between what you did and "the real McCoy," but there are also a whole series of differences that are critical to the proper conduct of this therapy. For example, a very real part of SRT is the need to restrict the amount of sleep time one gets for a few weeks. The idea here is to use sleep loss to ensure that people have the experience of falling asleep quickly. As prescribed by your physician, you'll have been able to rack up up to 7.5 hours of sleep. This is not likely to produce the kind of sleep loss needed to produce short sleep latencies or high sleep efficiency.

The bottom line here is that while well intentioned, what your physician had you do is not the standard form of treatment; not the form of therapy that has been studied in clinical trials and shown to have good effectiveness. That's why you're here—to get the "real McCoy" from one of the McCoys.

Patient: So I did part of the treatment, but not all of it?

Therapist: Right. It sounds like the forms of treatment you engaged in are indeed pretty much what we'll do here. But there are several critical differences.

The differences include:

- Minor changes in the treatment protocols so they better suit your case.
- Treatment will be conducted in a guided and supervised way. That is, we will work closely with you to make sure you're doing what you're supposed to do and when you're supposed to do it. Sort of like having a physical therapist or trainer, someone who works with you to help you accomplish what might otherwise be too difficult.

- Our form of treatment will be "data driven." That is, we'll take weekly measures so that we know precisely "how you're doing" and can make changes to your treatment only on the "force of data."

Bottom Line: Think of insomnia as a wall that you need to get over and beyond. With good intentions, someone said, "I know what you need—you need a ladder." And they were right; you do need a ladder. But instead of giving you a ladder, they gave you two rails and some rungs. And you did the best you could putting the ladder together. But the problem is that you only had a couple of rungs, and the rungs were spaced close together at the bottom. So you got off the ground, but didn't have enough distance to clear the wall. My job is to provide more rungs and to space the rungs just so.

Concerns About Sleep Restriction and Stimulus Control

Much of the resistance to procedures like sleep restriction and stimulus control stem from fears about the effects that such sleep deprivation will have during daytime. Questions about stamina, productivity, and illness will arise in much the same way that was discussed with regard to fears about reducing sleep medications. Therefore, the strategies employed to break down resistance to medication reduction can be utilized here and need not be elaborated again. However, there are some unique concerns that are raised by these procedures and will usually need to be addressed at some point in the therapy.

As always, the keys to reducing resistance will involve providing a good rationale for the techniques to be employed and making sure that the patient develops a positive expectation about what will occur. Once this has been done it is likely that patient will have many questions regarding how best to carry out these procedures. With regard to sleep restriction and stimulus control, a good deal of time may need to be spent on how the patient can remain awake for long hours in the evening that are sometimes required by these interventions.

Dialogue #41: There Is No Way I Can Stay Up That Late!

Patient: How am I ever going to stay up until two in the morning? There's no way I can stay up that late.

Therapist: Have you ever been awake until two in the morning?

Patient: Well yes I suppose so, like for New Year's Eve, but that's different. I was occupied with "partying like it was 1999," which in fact was the last time I did this.

Therapist: I think you just hit the nail on the head. One of the things that made this possible, aside from the fact that you were younger, is that you were "occupied." So one answer to your question "How am I ever going to stay up until two in the morning?" is to plan for as much activity in the evening as you possibly can.

Patient: Yes but there are only so many activities I can reasonably be expected to do in the evening night after night.

Therapist: True, but still it may help to make a list of things you can do in the evening. Some of this may require planning. For instance, you may want to rent several movies, purchase new games for the computer, or purchase the materials to start a new art project. The important thing here is to identify stuff that will make the time pass and the experience relatively enjoyable—this and to make sure that you're not caught later with nothing to do and feeling sleepy, or literally sleeping, on the sofa.

Patient: That's all well and good, but I still don't think I can be that active every night. And some of those things you suggest, like watching movies are likely to put me to sleep anyway.

Therapist: Fair enough. There will be times when it is unavoidable to feel sleepy, but there are still steps you can take to ensure that you will remain awake. When sitting, make sure to sit forward on chair or sofa, so that if you begin to fall sleep, it will startle you and wake you up. When you reach a point where you're falling asleep while sitting, then stand up and perhaps put some cold water on your face and neck. These steps should have the desired effect of allowing you to sit down for a while longer. But if you then feel sleepy again, simply repeat the steps and this should be enough to get you to your scheduled bedtime.

Patient: I can't live my life like that; it's crazy!

Therapist: I know it seems crazy. Try to remember this is a short-term "gig." No one expects you to live your life like this. Remember that as your sleep becomes more solid we will expand the amount of time you spend in bed. As you get more sleep with greater efficiency, we expect that you will feel less sleepy in the evening and of course you will eventually have an earlier bedtime. Remember that there is a light at the end of the tunnel.

Patient: Couldn't I just go to bed couple of hours earlier and see what happens?

Therapist: Haven't you done that in the past?

Patient: Yes

Therapist: And what was the result?

Patient: Well I guess I usually wake up more often or wake too early in the morning and can't get back to sleep.

Therapist: So going to bed earlier usually doesn't work for you. So let's try it our way for a few weeks.

Patient: Okay. I guess.

Therapist: One final irony here I'd like you to take note of. When you first came for help with your sleep, your complaint was that you couldn't fall asleep. Now what do we find ourselves talking about? The fact that "you can't stay awake." Ironic huh? We must be on the right track, eh?

Patient: (Laugh) I guess.

6
A Case Example*

Date of Evaluation. July 7, 2004

Identifying Information. Samuel Busch is a 62-year-old, married, Euro-American male who works part time as a financial consultant. He and his wife have a 29-year-old son and a 31-year-old daughter. He is 5'10" and weighs 190 lbs (Body Mass Index = 27.3).

PRESENTING COMPLAINT AND SLEEP INFORMATION

Presenting Complaint. "I have had trouble falling asleep since college. It's been pretty bad lately and I am afraid it will prevent me from returning to work full-time."

Daytime Functioning/Symptoms. Mr. Busch reportedly wakes up with a dry mouth and headaches 1 to 2 mornings per week. He stated that his daytime fatigue interferes with his ability to work and enjoy daily activities. He expressed a specific concern that his problems with insomnia might interfere with his plans to return to a full-time work schedule.

History of Presenting Complaint. Mr. Busch first experienced insomnia when in college and has been intermittently bothered by sleep initiation and maintenance problems since then (0–3 nights weekly). He indicated that he tolerated his sleep difficulties, which flared periodically during times of stress, until 2001. At this time, his sleep initiation problem worsened in association with some job-related turmoil (Mr. Busch was a Corporate VP in an organization that was in the midst of a massive "downsizing"). In response to the demands of his job, he began working late into the night

---

* **NOTE:** This case example is not drawn from an individual case and as such does not represent any one patient. The name used to identify the patient in the case example is fictitious. The report itself is longer than might be written for a typical clinical practice. The breadth of this review is intended to serve an educational purpose.

and attempted to cope with daytime fatigue by drinking large quantities of caffeine (9 cups–15 cups a day) during the week days and by sleeping late on the weekends. In 2002, his contract was not renewed, reportedly because of the corporate restructuring. In 2003, he experienced a second significant life stressor when his wife was diagnosed with uterine cancer. At this time, he gained 30 lbs. (from 190 lbs to 220 lbs) and his insomnia worsened to the point where it was a significant problem every night. He first sought evaluation and treatment for sleep disturbance at that time.

Prior Treatment for Sleep Disorders. In February 2002, Mr. Busch was evaluated by Dr. Pickwick at the Dickens' Sleep Disorders Center, Atlanta, Georgia. He sought help at this time, at the urging of his wife who complained that he was snoring excessively at night. In addition to trouble initiating and maintaining sleep, he reported that, at this time, he experienced severe daytime sleepiness in addition to fatigue. He underwent a PSG study and the results indicated mild obstructive sleep apnea (Respiratory Disturbance Index [RDI] 10 per hour). No evidence of other intrinsic sleep disorders was obtained. Treatment recommendations were to lose weight and to use nightly CPAP (a form of ventilation, which increases the patency of the oropharyngeal airway during sleep). Mr. Busch reportedly lost 25 pounds, with noticeable improvement in snoring and daytime sleepiness, but he still reported trouble falling and staying asleep. He reportedly did not tolerate the CPAP device, which he stated made his insomnia "way worse."

After discontinuing CPAP, he sought treatment from his primary care physician (PCP) who worked with Mr. Busch to cut back on caffeine and attend to sleep hygiene issues. He no longer drinks coffee after 12 noon and he exercises regularly 3 times a week for 30–60 minutes per occasion. His PCP also prescribed amitriptyline 20 mg, qhs. Mr. Busch reported that this medication provided some benefit as it allowed him to fall asleep more quickly. He was also less troubled by middle of the night awakenings, and according to his wife, the medication made his snoring less severe.

Unfortunately these gains were accompanied by anti-cholinergic effects (chronically swollen parotid glands with occasional flares of swelling as seen with "Wind Parotitis"). These side effects were not tolerable for the patient and he discontinued the amitriptyline after 3 months. Mr. Busch has since tried, and benefited from, temazepam and zolpidem. Neither he nor his PCP, however, wish to use these medications on a long-term basis. At present, he has discontinued all medications from the fear of becoming addicted. In June of 2004, Mr. Busch was re-referred to Dr. Pickwick for his problems with persistent insomnia. After physical exam and a repeat PSG study [which revealed that the RDI was within normal limits (4/hour)], Dr. Pickwick referred the patient to the Behavioral Sleep Medicine Service for evaluation and treatment.

Sleep Continuity/Quality. In the past 6 months, Mr. Busch reported trouble falling asleep with a sleep latency of 90 to 120 minutes, 4 or more nights per week, including weekends. Although his sleep latency reportedly varies from night to night, he reports that he rarely falls asleep in less than 30 minutes. He also indicated that he wakes up 2 to 3 times per night for about 30 to 60 minutes total, approximately 4 nights per week. He denied early morning awakenings. He reported getting an average of 5 hours to 6 hours of sleep per night.

Of note is that Mr. Busch states that when attempting to fall asleep or return to sleep, he ruminates and feels cognitively aroused ("can't turn my mind off") despite feeling tired and fatigued during the day. His thought content is often focused on current concerns. He also worries about how well he is about to sleep. In addition, when he awakens in the middle of the night he reports that he feels angry about his sleeplessness and is worried about his next-day's work performance. When sleeping in novel environments (work travel or vacations), Mr. Busch reports his insomnia is reliably less severe under these conditions. Finally, Mr. Busch indicated that he often has trouble waking up on time, and that if allowed, he can sleep late into the morning (late equals up to 8:30 AM).

Sleep Habits and Environment. Mr. Busch sleeps with his wife in a king size, pillow-top bed. The mattress and pillows are less than 3 years old. He currently maintains a preferred sleep phase of approximately 10:00 PM to 6:00 AM, adjusting this to 1:00 AM to 8:00 AM on the weekends. His wife goes to sleep at an earlier time (9:00 PM) and awakens earlier than Mr. Busch (5:30 AM) to be on time for work. His wife has told him that he sleeps restlessly and moves around a lot at night. Mr. Busch indicated that his sleep environment is comfortable but is not well light and sound attenuated (the room does not remain dark after sunrise). The bedroom temperature is kept relatively warm. He reports watching television and reading in bed. He reports that he sleeps with a radio at night for the "white noise" that it produces since he is awakened easily by outside noises. He no longer drinks coffee after noon. Mr. Busch drinks two martinis a night, three on special occasions. This pattern has been invariant since his late 40s. He denies using alcohol as a sedative (to help him fall asleep or stay asleep). The patient reports quitting tobacco use 10 years ago (smoked 1 ppd for 32 years).

He reports his mealtimes are regular with dinner around 7 PM, and occasionally has a snack before bed. He then "unwinds" by watching CNN, working, or making various job search and career plans. He will typically begin his bedtime routine around 9:00 PM. Around the time his wife falls asleep (9:30) he will get into bed and turn the television on. He doesn't feel like he "tries" to initiate sleep until about 10:00 PM. He reports that despite excessive daytime sleepiness he seldom is able to initiate naps and as a result does not attempt to nap more than once per month on a Sunday afternoon.

FAMILY AND SOCIAL HISTORY

The patient lives with his wife of 34 years. They have two children who are ages 29 (male) and 31 (female), who are healthy and independent young adults. Mr. Busch is an only child. Both parents have been deceased for 10 years, having died from cardiovascular disease. His father was a prominent attorney who he described as a "workaholic" who frequently complained of insomnia, but never sought treatment. His mother worked as a part-time nurse. Mr. Busch denied any family psychiatric history. The patient stated that he enjoyed a relatively happy childhood with no reported history of physical or sexual abuse. Mr. Busch characterized himself as having been a hard driving student as teenager who was active in sports. He graduated at the top of his high school class before earning his BA at The University of Pennsylvania and his MBA degree from The Wharton School. He met his wife in graduate school. Mr. Busch characterized the marriage as "better than most," "better than most people hope for or even imagine. . . ." His wife's diagnosis with cancer was characterized as "the worst thing that ever happened to him," but that he is optimistic that she is "on the mend." Mrs. Busch is status post-hysterectomy and appears in good health.

MEDICAL AND PSYCHIATRIC INFORMATION

Medical History. The patient denied any perinatal complications, reportedly achieved all developmental milestones within the normal time frames and described himself as having a relatively "healthy childhood" with the exception of frequent throat infections which abated following a tonsillectomy (1950). The patient's adult medical history is significant for a closed head injury with loss of consciousness (1960); chronic lower back and lower extremity musculoskeletal pain (since High School) [Mr. Busch believes these problems are secondary to sports injuries sustained playing intramural basketball in college]; frequent heartburn (GERD), particularly after rich meals, without reported nocturnal sequelae (since 1975); moderate-chronic Irritable Bowel Syndrome (w/o findings on colonoscopy [since 2000]); gall bladder disease (1995). His mild chronic pain condition is managed well with ibuprofen, prn. His gastroesphageal reflux disease is treated with daily doses of ranitidine. The Irritable Bowel Syndrome (IBS) is only a problem during periods of stress and is not currently being treated. The gall bladder disease was successfully treated with a cholecystectomy (1995).

Current Medications. Ranitidine 75 mg (daily), ibuprofen 600 mg, prn (2 days / week for back pain).

Psychiatric History. Mr. Busch denied psychiatric or psychological treatment, including hospitalizations. He also denied a history of suicidal ideation or attempts. Based on his self-report, it is likely that he experienced

a significant adjustment disorder with depressed mood after the loss of his corporate position in 2002 and with the diagnosis of his wife's cancer in 2003.

Mental Status Exam. The patient was a well-groomed and distinguished looking gentleman. He presented carrying a leather briefcase, wearing khaki pants, and a button down shirt, while holding a cup of coffee. His speech was normal in volume, rate, and tone. He was pleasant and cooperative. His affect was euthymic, appropriate to content and full in range. He described his mood as "ok, but somewhat irritable." He appeared to be mildly self-critical. Mr. Busch denied current and past suicidal/homicidal ideation, intent, or plan. He denied any specific fears or phobias, but admitted that he has always been somewhat of a worrier and that under stress he can worry up to 50% of the day. However, when not under pressure his worrying often abates. His thought contents were focused on presenting his symptoms with no evidence of bizarre or delusional beliefs. Mr. Busch was oriented to person, place, and time. His thought processes were logical and goal directed with no distractibility noted. His insight, judgment, and impulse control appeared to be good. His intellect appeared to be well above average, although his IQ was not formally assessed.

SUMMARY OF RESULTS FROM ASSESSMENT MEASURES

As part of the intake evaluation, Mr. Busch was administered eight instruments which specifically assay information related to sleep and mood. This information is presented below and quantifies the patient's sleep complaints, "flags" occult mood disturbance, and quantifies the patient's pretreatment status.

INSTRUMENT	MEASURE OF	SCORE RANGE	PATIENT'S SCORE
ISI[1]	Severity of insomnia	0–28	19
PSQI[2]	Sleep disturbance	0–21	15
ESS[3]	Daytime sleepiness	0–24	9
KSS[4]	Daytime sleepiness	0–9	6
MFI[5]	General fatigue	0–20	12
	Physical fatigue	0–20	10
	Reduced activity	0–20	14
	Reduced motivation	0–20	12
	Mental fatigue	0–20	17
BDI[6]	Depression	0–63	10

STAI[7]	Anxiety	0–80	40
POMS (SF)[8]	Total Score	0–145	57
	1. Tension/anxiety	0–25	18
	2. Depression/dejection	0–25	7
	3. Anger/hostility	0–25	18
	4. Vigor	0–25	12
	5. Fatigue	0–25	13
	6. Confusion	0–20	9

1. ISI—	Insomnia Severity Scale	2. PSQI—	The Pittsburgh Sleep Inventory
3. ESS—	The Epworth Sleepiness Scale	4. KSS—	The Karolinska Sleepiness Scale
5. MFI—	The Multidimenoinal Fatigue Inventory	6. BDI—	The Beck Depression Inventory
7. STAI—	The State Trait Anxiety Inventory	8. POMS—	The Profile of Mood States

The data acquired from these instruments are consistent with the clinical interview. Mr. Busch exhibits moderately severe sleep disturbance and insomnia, moderate to high levels of sleepiness (relative to insomnia norms), and moderate fatigue—which is most evident and severe on measures of mental fatigue. Of particular importance is that both sleepiness measures (along with a Hx of OSA) suggest that the patient may be at risk, given the side effects of CBT-I, for substantially worse excessive daytime sleepiness during treatment.

Within the mood domain, Mr. Busch appears to exhibit more anxiety (STAI) than depression (BDI) and this result is paralleled on the POMS with high scores on scales 1 and 3. While none of the mood scores fall within the pathologic range, the values are close enough to the clinical cutoffs to warrant attention.

CASE CONCEPTUALIZATION

Socioeconomic and Cultural Factors. From a broad perspective, Mr. Busch's complaint can be conceptualized as growing out of a societal devaluation of the importance of sleep and the hyper-valuation of productivity. It can be argued that these prevailing sentiments loom larger in the corporate climate where Mr. Busch functioned as a top executive. In this environment, working late into the night is the norm. Fatigue and the effects of sleep deprivation are routinely minimized and many of the compensatory behaviors used to ameliorate such effects, while romanticized, directly contribute to the development of chronic insomnia (e.g., chronic use of stimulants, irregular sleep wake schedules, the use of alcohol as a hypnotic, etc.). In short, it is likely that the cultural back drop, including Mr. Busch's own family of origin's "subculture," have substantially contributed to the clinical course of his sleep disorder.

Social and Behavioral Factors. Mr. Busch described several factors that are consistent with the potential role of modeling and classical conditioning in

the maintenance of his insomnia. With respect to modeling, it appears that Mr. Busch has adopted an approach to work and life consistent with the model of role functioning provided by his father. He learned at an early age to place an extreme degree of importance on work and performance at the expense of maintaining a well-balanced life style. Mr. Busch's father (presumably his primary male role model) reportedly sacrificed a consistent daily routine and regular sleep/wake schedule to pursue career success. As indicated above, his father also suffered from insomnia. While a chronic problem, Mr. Busch's father did not seek medical attention and this may have conveyed the message that sleeplessness was/is not to be considered a significant problem. Consistent with this conceptualization is that Mr. Busch only sought treatment at the insistence of his wife, some 40 years after his problems first manifested.

With respect to the potential role of conditioning, his presentation is consistent with a number of factors that point to the possibility that conditioned hyperarousal may play a central role in maintaining his chronic insomnia complaint. Mr. Busch noted that despite feeling fatigued during the day, he feels alert and ruminative when it is time for bed, suggesting that the bed and bedroom operate as conditioned stimuli eliciting cognitive arousal that interferes with sleep initiation and maintenance. Further evidence of a discriminative, learned association of arousal with his bed and bedroom is suggested by Mr. Busch's observation that when he sleeps in a new environment, such as a hotel room, he has less trouble sleeping. Mr. Busch also described a common complaint among patients with primary insomnia, i.e., pre-sleep thought content focused on his inability to fall asleep and stay asleep and on the potential consequences of poor sleep on his career. Such negative cognitions can lead to performance anxiety and may become readily conditioned to the pre-sleep state.

Life Events. Life stressors appear to have played an important role in initiating Mr. Busch's chronic sleep problems. His original acute episodes of insomnia were likely precipitated by a combination of a Phase Delay and stress associated with scholastic life and/or final exams in college. The insomnia, which is now chronic, is likely to have been precipitated (as a chronic disorder) by the events that occurred in 2001 through 2003. As previously indicated, during this time Mr. Busch experienced a significant increase in stress at work, the development of poor sleep hygiene in association with work-related stress (e.g., working late into the night, increasing caffeine consumption, decreasing physical exercise, and extending his sleep period on weekends), significant weight gain, and ultimately the loss of his high paying, high status corporate vice presidency. The stress of his wife's cancer diagnosis also appears to have been a significant "precipitating factor" for the insomnia to the extent that it did not allow Mr. Busch time to recover from the stressors of the prior two years.

Genetics and Temperament. Mr. Busch described some traits which appear to make him particularly susceptible to physiologic hyper-reactivity and/or hyperarousal. He described himself as having a hard-driving, perfectionist, achievement-oriented personality style. He stated that he often "overreacts" to minor stressors and he generally has trouble physically "winding down" after becoming aggravated. Mr. Busch also described himself as "hyper" and joked that he must have the "metabolic rate of a chipmunk." Finally, he characterized himself as a "worrier." Each of these characterizations represent or correspond to forms of arousal that are likely to contribute to insomnia (as well as other stress-related conditions like GERD, Irritable Bowel Syndrome, and chronic musculoskeletal pain). Finally, Mr. Busch appears to have a predisposition for Delayed Sleep Phase Disorder as evidenced by his tendency (both as a young adult and now) to delay his sleep period on the weekends.

OVERALL CONCEPTUALIZATION

Mr. Busch's chronic insomnia may be understood broadly from within the context of the behavioral model of Insomnia (aka the Spielman Model or the 3 Factor Model of Insomnia).

Mr. Busch exhibits a variety of characteristics that may be identified as predisposing factors including hyper-reactivity, somatic hyperarousal and a tendency toward worry and rumination. Each of these factors is likely to make Mr. Busch vulnerable to insomnia, particularly during times of stress. Mr. Busch reported a variety of incidences that may be identified as precipitating factors including, although not limited to, the events that lead up to the loss of his job and his wife's illness. Finally, Mr. Busch engaged in a variety of behaviors that may be characterized as "perpetuating factors" which were/are implemented to compensate for insomnia and daytime fatigue. Rather than correct the problem, these strategies serve to maintain the insomnia (in the absence of the original precipitating factors) and/or contribute to the development of conditioned hyperarousal that is characteristic of chronic insomnia. Mr. Busch engaged in a number of maladaptive strategies such as sleeping in on weekends, drinking excessive amounts of caffeine, and spending excessive time awake in bed in an effort to obtain more sleep, etc. Each of these strategies disrupt the homeostatic and circadian regulation of sleep and increase the opportunity for the bed and bedroom to become classically conditioned stimuli for wakefulness. Evidence for the presence of conditioned arousal in Mr. Busch's case is suggested by his report of improved sleep when in a different environment (change in conditioned stimuli) as well as his reported experiencing of an abrupt increase in cognitive arousal (mind racing, etc) when he lays down to sleep.

DIAGNOSIS AND RECOMMENDATIONS

Diagnostic Impression:

Mr. Busch clearly meets criteria for Primary Insomnia. He also exhibits a tendency toward excessive worry that may or may not be strictly stress-related. At this time, it is not apparent that worry limits his ability to function well during the day. His tendency toward worry and his anxiety symptoms will be monitored over the course of treatment so that we may better assess whether the patient has a diagnosable anxiety disorder. Finally, we will want to continue to assess whether he has a true phase delay.

Axis I: 307.42 Primary Insomnia
309.28 H/O Adjustment disorder with mixed anxious and depressed mood

r/o as co-morbid or contributory factors:
—Circadian Factors (Phase Delay);
—Generalized Anxiety Disorder

Axis II: Deferred
Axis III: Low Back Pain, GERD, IBS, H/O OSA

Axis IV: Loss of CEO position in 2002 and only Consultant work since. Wife diagnosed with Cancer in 2003.

Axis V: Current GAF: 61

NOTE: For pedagogical purposes this section will be specifically focused on applying our algorhythm to determine if Mr. Busch is a candidate for CBT-I.

30/30 DIMS
Does the PT take ≥30 min to fall asleep   Yes
Is the PT awake for ≥30 min during the night   Yes
Does the patient have a daytime complaint related to this insomnia   Yes

PHASE
The 30/30 DIMS problems exist with ad libitum sleep schedule   Yes

Comment: There is both a history and a current practice where the patient phase delays his preferred sleep schedule. This not with standing the patient still exhibits DIMS problems.

UNDX—or—UNTX ILLNESS
Does the patient have an undiagnosed (UNDX),   Yes
untreated (UNTX) medical and/or psychiatric illness.

Comment: The patient may have an undiagnosed anxiety disorder but as evaluated here there is not enough data to make a firm diagnosis. Even if, however, the patient had, e.g., GAD, this would not necessarily contraindicate the use of CBT-I. More important is whether the anxiety disorder would interfere with, or be made worse by, CBT-I.

UNSTABLE ILLNESS

Does the patient have an unstable or unresolved medical   Yes
and/or psychiatric illness

Comment: It can be conservatively argued that the patient's GERD, IBS and Low Back Pain constitute unresolved medical problems. Again, the issue is whether the unstable illness would interfere with or be made worse by CBT-I.

ASSESS

Is it possible the insomnia will resolve with the acute illness?   No

Comment: Mr. Busch's medical conditions may be considered as unresolved medical conditions—conditions which occur periodically. Because the insomnia is persistent and severe, and the IBS, GERD and Low Back Pain are episodic, it seems clear that the insomnia is occurring independent of these conditions. This said, if the other conditions were also persistent and severe, there is still enough evidence to suggest that CBT-I is indicated on the basis of the existence of clear behavioral factors (perpetuating factors). More aggressive treatment for each of the medical conditions may nonetheless be warranted and contribute to a better treatment response to CBT-I.

ASSESS

Do the illnesses prevent the patient from engaging in SRT or SCT?   No

ASSESS

Will SRT or SCT aggravate the "co-morbid" Illness?   No

Comment: It is possible that the sleep loss from SRT or SCT will aggravate the IBS, GERD and/or Low Back Pain. In the absence of any substantial data on such subjects, it is best to assume that treatment might exacerbate these conditions—but do so on a temporary basis. Accordingly, CBT-I treatment is not contraindicated, but it may be best to plan for how to manage mild to moderate worsening of these other symptoms during treatment.

LOW SLEEP EFFICIENCY

Does the patient have an SE < 90%
(Is there evidence of maladaptive behaviors?)   Yes

Final Assessment: CBT-I is indicated for this patient.

TREATMENT PLAN

Gather one week of sleep continuity data prospectively with sleep diaries. Provided that these data are consistent with Mr. Busch's presenting complaints, use the data from this baseline period to establish the parameters for Sleep Restriction Therapy (SRT). Along with SRT, deploy stimulus control, sleep hygiene, and cognitive therapy according to our clinic's standard treatment regimen. Measure EDS symptoms weekly to insure that these are not exacerbated by therapy to a degree that puts the patient at risk for accidents, injury or non-adherence.

Issues for Follow Up:

1. Provide Mr. Busch's PCP with a copy of this report and determine if there is any reason not to proceed with treatment. That is, barring issues pertaining to interactions with medications or medical conditions, is this a good time for Mr. Busch to pursue treatment?

2. Given that Mr. Busch exhibited a degree of Circadian dysrhythmia, if adequate treatment gains are not forthcoming and the phase delay symptoms persist or worsen, consider the use of bright light therapy.

3. Evaluate Mr. Busch's mood status during the course of treatment. If adequate treatment gains are not forthcoming and the anxiety symptoms persist or worsen, consider a referral for assessment and treatment of the apparent anxiety disorder.

4. Evaluate Mr. Busch's medical conditions (pain, GERD, IBS). If adequate treatment gains are not forthcoming and these symptoms persist or worsen, consider a referral for assessment and treatment of these disorders.

5. Following treatment, if Mr. Busch's insomnia has resolved and he exhibits EDS or develops the complaint of nonrestorative sleep, consider a reevaluation of his OSA and refer for PSG.

BEHAVIORAL SLEEP MEDICINE SERVICE—PROGRESS NOTE

Name: S. Busch
Session 2:   Review Baseline Sleep Diary Data; Initiate SRT & SCT

CPT Code:

90804	90806	90847	90853

Medications: Ranitidine 75 mg. Daily   **Adherence:**   Yes ☒
Ibuprofen 600 PRN   Partial
No

TTB:	10:00 pm
SOL:	75 min.
FNA:	3.5
WASO:	121 min.
TST:	336 min.
TIB:	532 min.
TOB:	6:57 am
SE:	63%

Fatigue	+	DSPS/ASPS	?	Appetite	–
Dozing/Naps	+	SI/HI	–	Interest	–
Concentration	+	Nightmares	–	Mood	–

ESS	6
BDI	8
STAI	40

+	Clinically Relevant
–	Clinically not relevant
SI-	Suicidal Ideation
HI–	Homicidal Ideation

Subjective/Issues: Mr. Busch reported that his diaries were "pretty consistent" with his typical sleep pattern, except this week he seemed to be awake for more time in the middle of the night. He denied napping but did admit to dozing on the sofa in the evenings. Mr. Busch's sense was that these episodes rarely last more than a few minutes and that they signal that it is time for him to go to bed. He confided that he was eager to get underway with treatment but also felt a bit nervous about what he might have to do. He denied any other current worry or anxiety, which somewhat mitigates our concerns about the possibility of co-morbid GAD.

Treatment: The patient was oriented to our clinic's standard form of SCT and SRT. It was decided based on the week's prior sleep diary data that time in bed (TIB) would be set at 5.5 hrs. Given Mr. Busch's preferences for a work week schedule and a schedule that is also more compatible with his wife's preferred sleep phase, an early rise time was adopted (6:00 am). Since TIB was set to 5.5 hours this allowed for a prescribed Time to Bed (TTB) of 12:30 am. Despite the preference for this schedule during the work week, Mr. Busch balked at the idea of having to get up early on the weekends. He acquiesced when it was explained that the sleep schedule we were establishing was temporary and was geared to produce clinical gains during treatment. He seemed greatly comforted by the thought that sometime in the future he would again be able to "sleep in" on the weekends. While we did not disabuse him of this idea, his tendency for phase delay may make it likely that even with the successful resolution of his Primary Insomnia, he may not be able to tolerate regular and/or large phase shifts. This issue may need to be revisited later in treatment.

As part of "planning for SCT and SRT" we discussed at length what activities Mr. Busch should engage in during the phase delay in his TTB and during the night while he practices SCT. He expressed an interest in doing work at these times. While such activities may be rewarding, if not pleasant to Mr. Busch, I expressed the concern that accomplishing significant amounts of work during the desired sleep period may, in the short run, help him "while away the time" but that in the long run such behaviors may reinforce the insomnia by 1) giving the problem "a positive function" and 2) increasing the tendency of work stress to produce insomnia. Thus, it was best for him engage in enjoyable, non-work related activities. Mr. Busch's second idea about how to spend his "new found time" was to play video games—a "skill" recently taught to him by his 5 year old grandson. He reported that the activity is very engaging and the idea of practicing so that he can eventually "whip" his grandson held enormous appeal, so much so that he went on to express concern about staying up too long. I reminded him that the goal was to build up "pressure for sleep" and that "staying up too long" would in fact be just fine.

Given Mr. Busch's scores on the ESS, BDI, and the STAI, it is important to monitor these over time. A sustained increase in symptom severity of 50% or more for 2 or more weeks should, for the purposes of this case, be considered cause for the consideration of a targeted intervention.

Date: 7/21/04   **RTC:** 7/28/04   **Signature**

BEHAVIORAL SLEEP MEDICINE SERVICE—PROGRESS NOTE

Name: S. Busch
Session 3: Adjust SCT & SRT

CPT Code:

90804	90806	90847	90853

Medications: Ranitidine 75 mg. Daily   **Adherence:**   Yes **X**
Ibuprofen 600 PRN   Partial
                                                              No

TTB:	12:30 am
SOL:	50.5 min.
FNA:	2.7
WASO:	22.8 min.
TST:	256 min.
TIB:	330 min.
TOB:	6:05 am
SE:	77.5%

Fatigue	+	DSPS/ASPS	?	Appetite	−
Dozing/Naps	+	SI/HI	−	Interest	−
Concentration	+	Nightmares	−	Mood	−

ESS	7
BDI	5
STAI	35

Subjective/Issues: Mr. Busch complained from the outset that he didn't know if he could do this much longer. He felt that he hadn't made substantial gains over the course of the week and that his daytime fatigue was worse than ever—to a point where he actually felt sleepy during the day. I reminded him of our discussion regarding the notion that he would get worse before getting better—and pointed out that he had in fact improved: his SL and WASO had decreased. As an exercise to underscore this point, we calculated the percent improvement for these variables and for his sleep efficiency. He admitted that his sleep continuity numbers appeared to be moving in the right direction, and further he acknowledged that the increase in fatigue was something that was predicted at the last session. We discussed ways to combat the emergent fatigue (including outdoor walks, the judicious use of caffeine, phototherapy, and/or the use of a prescription stimulants for the first few weeks of therapy). Mr. Busch seemed glad to hear that there were some alternatives but felt that at this point he'd "tough it out".

Areas of concern center on the fact that the patient admits to still falling asleep on the sofa before bedtime, and that he is not consistently getting out of bed for awakenings that occur after sleep onset. The former is explained by the idea that he just can't stay awake, and the latter by the idea that he sometimes feels that if he just waits in bed longer that he will eventually fall asleep. Each of these issues were discussed. Ways of staying awake until the prescribed bedtime were reviewed. If these aspects of compliance continue to be problematic, we'll consider monitoring him with actigraphy. This will provide not only some additional data regarding his sleep continuity but—more importantly—a means towards measuring compliance.

Treatment Plan: Given that Mr. Busch did not reach the target SE of 90%, we did not recommend that he upwardly titrate his TIB. Conversely, we did not downwardly titrate TIB due to his noncompliance with stimulus control. Although disappointed that he will not be able to sleep more yet, he seemed pleased enough with his progress that he'd be willing to "give it a shot" for another week. As indicated above, most of this session was spent working on problem solving in the service of compliance. Sleep hygiene will be covered in the next session since time did not allow for it in this session.

Date: 7/28/04   **RTC:** 8/4/04   **Signature** _____

BEHAVIORAL SLEEP MEDICINE SERVICE—PROGRESS NOTE

Name: S. Busch
Session 4: Adjust SCT & SRT; Sleep Hygiene

CPT Code:

90804	90806	90847	90853

Medications: Ranitidine 75 mg. Daily   **Adherence:**   Yes **X**
Ibuprofen 600 PRN   Partial
                                              No

TTB:	12:30 am
SOL:	8.5 min.
FNA:	1.1
WASO:	10 min.
TST:	311 min.
TIB:	330 min.
TOB:	6:00 am
SE:	94%

Fatigue	+	DSPS/ASPS	?	Appetite	−
Dozing/Naps	−	SI/HI	−	Interest	−
Concentration	+	Nightmares	−	Mood	+

ESS	12
BDI	13
STAI	55

Subjective/Issues: Despite the fact that Mr. Busch felt "bone tired" he is pleased by the fact that he is now both getting to sleep more quickly and when he wakes he is getting back to sleep quickly again. We both agreed that it is time to expand his sleep opportunity, but to do so carefully. With regard to sleep hygiene, the patient questioned why he needs to be concerned with these factors if he is already sleeping fairly solidly. He also reported that although he is still extremely sleepy in the evening, the strategies we discussed last session are working to prevent his dozing off on the sofa. He is also feeling excited today because he has been offered an opportunity to become the president of a fledgling R&D company. He admitted this will be stressful but also believes that it will be quite challenging and rewarding.

Treatment: Standard upward titration instructions were given so that starting tonight Mr. Busch can go to bed at 12:15am. He was cautioned to maintain strict regular hours and stimulus control. The rest of the session was spent on sleep hygiene. His question regarding the actual importance of sleep hygiene lead to a discussion of how maintaining good habits may not obviously make his sleep better now, but that as he expands sleep opportunity, good sleep habits can have impact on how much he can expand sleep opportunity, and make him less vulnerable to relapse in the future. After going over the list, the patient agreed to lower the bedroom temperature at night, replace radio noise with a more suitable white noise such as a fan. (Right now in summer his room AC will accomplish both of the first 2 points). He also agreed to restrict liquid intake to <7 oz. after 8:30 pm, and to have a light snack each night about 1 hr. prior to bedtime. He reluctantly agreed to decrease his alcohol consumption at night just as an experiment to see what effects this might have on improving his sleep. He will reduce his nightly consumption to one Martini per night. He also agreed to keep track of his alcohol use on his diaries. Finally, Mr. Busch did not feel that he can do much about light attenuating his bedroom at this point, because doing so would be either "too expensive or too much of a pain". He says he promised to revisit this issue again if it looks like it's a problem.

Finally it should be noted that patient exhibited an increase in sleepiness and mood symptomatology. This should be monitored accordingly.

Date: 8/4/04   **RTC:** 8/11/04   **Signature** _____

BEHAVIORAL SLEEP MEDICINE SERVICE—PROGRESS NOTE

Name: S. Busch
Session 5:   Adjust SCT and SRT

CPT Code:

90804	90806	90847	90853

Medications: Ranitidine 75 mg. Daily   **Adherence:**   Yes
Ibuprofen 600 PRN   Partial **X**
                                               No

TTB:	12:15 am
SOL:	6.5 min.
FNA:	0.7
WASO:	8.5 min.
TST:	330 min.
TIB:	345 min.
TOB:	6:00 am
SE:	95%

Fatigue	+	DSPS/ASPS	?	Appetite	−
Dozing/Naps	−	SI/HI	−	Interest	−
Concentration	+	Nightmares	−	Mood	−

ESS	9
BDI	10
STAI	45

Subjective/Issues: Mr. Busch volunteered that he is very pleased that his SE has held despite the increased time in bed. He wondered whether this will continue given his feeling that he will have to expand sleep opportunity quite a bit more in order to start feeling less tired during the day. He reported that he has been faithful to the sleep habit changes he agreed to last week, but has found it difficult to reduce his alcohol intake. This was true for two reasons. First, he is used to having two drinks per night. He indicated that he was successful "reigning this in" on all but one evening. The bigger problem is that he did in fact take the new job and that this entailed many dinner meetings with corporate executives who he characterized as "big time drinkers". At these meetings he allowed himself one drink per occasion and he explained that this is why he had more than one martini on several of the nights last week. Finally, he noted that the evening meetings were interfering with his exercise routine.

Treatment: Given that SE has held nicely, Mr. Busch was instructed to increase sleep opportunity by 15 min. This ongoing expansion of sleep opportunity continues to be proffered as an experiment in which we are trying to determine how these incremental changes in sleep opportunity will effect SE and ultimately daytime functioning. Given this frame of reference, Mr. Busch was encouraged to hold constant the other factors that might influence his sleep and only vary the behaviors and practices that we explicitly target with treatment. Since decreased alcohol use is part of the treatment regimen, time was spent on how to approach limiting his alcohol use to one drink per night for the next week or so. Finally, we revisited the issue of daytime fatigue and sleepiness and Mr. Busch indicated that he seemed to be functioning adequately, even though he was tired. It should be noted that sleepiness and mood scores were reduced. We will continue to monitor. We will introduce cognitive therapy next session.

Date: 8/11/04   **RTC:** 8/18/04   **Signature** _____

BEHAVIORAL SLEEP MEDICINE SERVICE—PROGRESS NOTE

Name: S. Busch
Session 6: Adjust SCT & SRT

CPT Code:

90804	90806	90847	90853

Medications: Ranitidine 75 mg. Daily   **Adherence:**   Yes
Ibuprofen 600 PRN   Partial **X**
                                      No

TTB:	12:00 am
SOL:	5 min.
FNA:	1.1
WASO:	49 min.
TST:	306 min.
TIB:	360 min.
TOB:	6:00 am
SE:	85%

Fatigue	+	DSPS/ASPS	?	Appetite	−
Dozing/Naps	−	SI/HI	−	Interest	−
Concentration	+	Nightmares	−	Mood	+

ESS	11
BDI	12
STAI	50

Subjective/Issues: Mr. Busch expressed some concern over his sleep this week. He reports that over the course of the last week he has tended to awaken about 30 mins. before his alarm. His experience of these early morning awakenings (EMAs) are that he is suddenly "wide awake" and is thinking about issues related to his new job. His response to the awakenings is to begin his day earlier; unfortunately, this has been associated with cat napping.

Treatment: The session focused on several items: 1. Issues related to "what constitutes good progress"; 2. The need to handle the EMAs differently; and 3. The association between "Cat Napping" on the couch and EMAs. Finally, because this session focused on the emergent events of the week, formal Cognitive Therapy for sleep related worry will be delayed until the next session. This along with last weeks issues make it likely that 1 additional session may be required.

1. Issues related to "what constitutes good progress". It was pointed out (using the chart graphs) that if there has been a setback—it has been a minor one as Mr. Busch's SOL and WASO are still reduced as compared to his baseline data and that his SE is still substantially higher (even on this bad week) then when he began treatment. This said, the reduction in SE was not substantial enough to warrant further upward titration this week. Mr. Busch initially responded to this by saying "I feel like your penalizing me for having a bad week". My response was that progress rarely occurs as we'd like it to—with a continuous upward trajectory. I asked if he could think of an analogy for when progress is still considered good progress even though there might be occasional setbacks. Mr. Busch drew an analogy to the stock market and the value of stock shares. Here things almost never move in a linear fashion: the line is always jagged—"2 steps up, 1 step down, no change, 2 steps up" type of progression. Mr. Busch seemed pleased with the analogy and comfortable leaving his sleep schedule unchanged for the next week.
2. The need to handle the EMAs differently. As covered in other sessions, we reminded Mr. Busch that it is not a good idea to give a function to an adverse event. That is, to potentially reinforce EMAs by allowing these events to be associated with good work productivity. We suggested that, as part of stimulus control, he should leave the bedroom, take some notes, and then retire to the bedroom again—where he relies on the alarm as the cue to start his day. If, however, he elects to just start his day—he needs to be extra vigilant about not "cat napping" on the couch on the following evening.
3. The association between "Cat Napping" on the couch and EMAs. As is so often the case, it was very easy to show Mr. Busch the temporal contiguity between his sleeping on the sofa and the occurrence of EMAs. We reviewed the issue in terms of the homeostatic regulation of sleep, and reminded Mr. Busch that "bleeding off the valve early in the night", may almost certainly guarantee either sleep initiation or maintenance problems.
We will continue to monitor sleepiness and mood symptoms.

Date: 8/18/04   **RTC:** 8/25/04   **Signature** _____

BEHAVIORAL SLEEP MEDICINE SERVICE—PROGRESS NOTE

Name: S. Busch
Session 7:   Adjust SCT and SRT

CPT Code: | 90804 | 90806 | 90847 | 90853 |

Medications: Ranitidine 75 mg. Daily   **Adherence**:   Yes
    Ibuprofen 600 PRN   Partial **X**
    No

TTB:	11:00 pm
SOL:	30 min.
FNA:	2.0
WASO:	52 min.
TST:	338 min.
TIB:	420 min.
TOB:	6:00 am
SE:	80%

Fatigue	+	DSPS/ASPS	?	Appetite	−
Dozing/Naps	−	SI/HI	−	Interest	−
Concentration	+	Nightmares	−	Mood	+

ESS	13
BDI	14
STAI	50

Subjective/Issues: Mr. Busch presented at today's session as very anxious and stated before our normal routine of crunching the numbers that " its all falling apart."

His diaries reflect that he advanced his bedtime by one hour and that he regularly showed delayed sleep onsets and on three occasions substantial EMAs. When queried about why he changed his sleep schedule "AMA"—he stated that that he needed to be up for work as it was a "make or break" week. To be up for the game he decided that he needed to get more sleep—to get more sleep he needed to go to bed earlier.

Treatment: In some way this setback represented a substantial opportunity. It allowed us to demonstrate—yet again—the "positive correlation fallacy". That is, more sleep opportunity does not necessarily mean more sleep. As important, this "unraveling" of the patient's gains allowed us to highlight that sleep related worry can precipitate bad judgments and lead to behaviors that, while well intended, lead to insomnia. This represented the perfect segue for us to engage in a round of cognitive therapy for catastrophic thoughts about the consequences of poor sleep. As might be expected, Mr. Busch's primary concerns were that poor sleep would lead to poor on the job performance. We were able to come up with a substantial list of possibilities and the consequences of such adverse events. On review of the items, it was easy to show the profound mismatch between Mr. Busch's certainty of negative outcomes and their vanishingly rare occurrence. The exercise was well received and Mr. Busch appeared ready and willing to resume the prescribed sleep schedule (12:00 am to 6:00 am).

Date: 8/25/04 **RTC:** 9/1/04 **Signature** _____

BEHAVIORAL SLEEP MEDICINE SERVICE—PROGRESS NOTE

Name: S. Busch
Session 8:   Adjust SCT & SRT

CPT Code:

90804	90806	90847	90853

Medications: Ranitidine 75 mg. Daily   **Adherence:**   Yes **X**
                   Ibuprofen 600 PRN   Partial
                                                                  No

TTB:	12:00 am
SOL:	7.5 min.
FNA:	1.0
WASO:	15 min.
TST:	337.5 min.
TIB:	360 min.
TOB:	6:00 am
SE:	93%

Fatigue	+	DSPS/ASPS	?	Appetite	−
Dozing/Naps	−	SI/HI	−	Interest	−
Concentration	+	Nightmares	−	Mood	−

ESS	9
BDI	10
STAI	40

Subjective/Issues: Mr. Busch reported "he's back in the saddle and—in keeping with the metaphor—things are going great guns". He reported that he feels like he is on the right track and is beginning to believe that he can sustain his forward momentum. His diaries reflected this in that his SLs were reliably short and that on three nights this week he slept until awakened by his alarm. (Note: The patient drew happy faces by these entries). When queried about why he thought he was successful with sleeping until the alarm, Mr. Busch admitted that in addition to getting back with the program (the prescribed sleep schedule & the practice of stimulus control) he decided to follow one of our prior recommendations—to purchase drapes for his bedroom. He reported being amazed that this made it so much easier to "sleep in".

Treatment: Mr. Busch is encouraged to keep up the good work, and given 93% SE is told to set bedtime 15 mins. earlier at 11:45. Cognitive work was also used to caution Mr. Busch not to expect perfect sleep every night, and that it may be unrealistic to think that he will get to a point when he never wakes early. In fact, time was taken to persuade him that that many good sleepers wake a few minutes before their alarms and that this represents not so much a problem as is a sign of a well entrained circadian rhythm.

Finally, Mr. Busch indicated that he needed to go on a business trip for 2 weeks and wondered if treatment could be delayed a few weeks. I explained that while the in-office sessions could be delayed, the treatment regimen needed to be continued. After some discussion, it was decided that Mr. Busch would adhere to the same schedule for the next two weeks—and not look to upwardly titrate his sleep opportunity until he got back.

Date: 9/8/04   **RTC:** 9/22/04   **Signature** _____

BEHAVIORAL SLEEP MEDICINE SERVICE—PROGRESS NOTE

Name: S. Busch

Session 9: Adjust SCT & SRT and Relapse Prevention

CPT Code:

90804	90806	90847	90853

Medications: Ranitidine 75 mg. Daily   **Adherence:** Yes **X**
Ibuprofen 600 PRN   Partial
                                           No

TTB:	11:45 pm
SOL:	6.5 min.
FNA:	0.5
WASO:	10 min.
TST:	358.5 min.
TIB:	375.0 min.
TOB:	6:00 am
SE:	95%

Fatigue	–	DSPS/ASPS	?	Appetite	–
Dozing/Naps	–	SI/HI	–	Interest	–
Concentration	+	Nightmares	–	Mood	–

ESS	7
BDI	5
STAI	35

Subjective/Issues: Mr. Busch returns after his two week trip feeling like he has "licked this problem." He states that during his travel, his sleep was no problem. His diaries reflect that he is waking with his alarm 2–3 nights/week and usually wakes 10–20 minutes early on other mornings. On the few occasions when he woke earlier, he practiced stimulus control. He is quite pleased that on those nights he no longer worries about sleep or work, and is becoming increasingly more confident that this will not lead to a pattern of poor sleep—if he does the right things.

Treatment: It is always difficult to know "where to go to from here". Should the patient continue upward titration? Should the patient continue stimulus control, etc. After some lengthy discussion, it was decided that Mr. Busch would leave his schedule fixed for the next 3 months and that he would continue to keep sleep diaries and practice stimulus control. If things do not continue to go well, he will implement another round of SRT on his own. In addition, he will continue to use the cognitive strategy we introduced to challenge negative expectations regarding sleep. We reviewed the rules and I encouraged him to drop me an email if he wished some input before the next round. Moreover, I reassured him that, if he felt he needed to go "back into training", I would provide him expedited access to our service. The balance of this session was focused on relapse prevention, i.e., what is a relapse, what to do in the event of an episode of insomnia, etc. Finally, it was suggested to him that, although his anxiety has decreased, his still elevated anxiety scores and his prior reactivity to stress suggest that he might benefit from a formal stress-management intervention which might include relaxation training. He was amenable to this notion and we provided him with some referral information.

Date: 9/22/04   **RTC:** Case Closed   **Signature** _____

Graphs for Mr. Busch's Progress Over the Course of Treatment

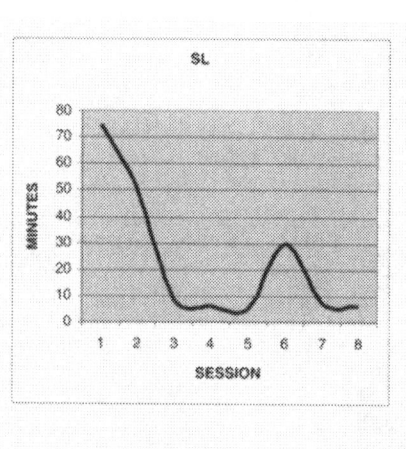

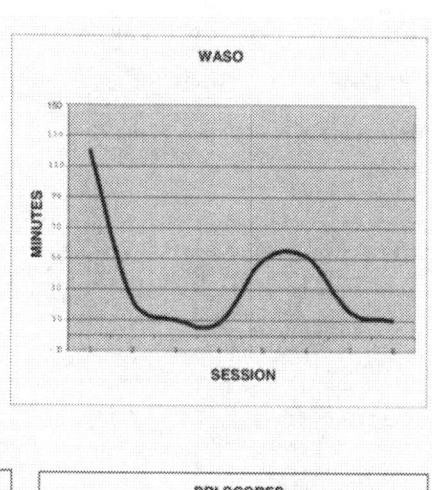

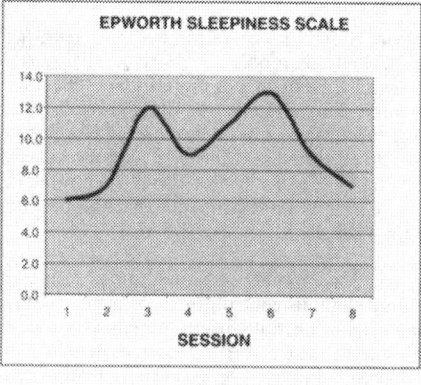

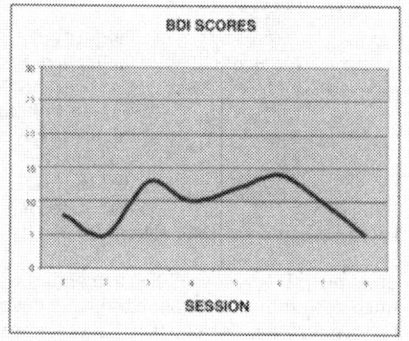

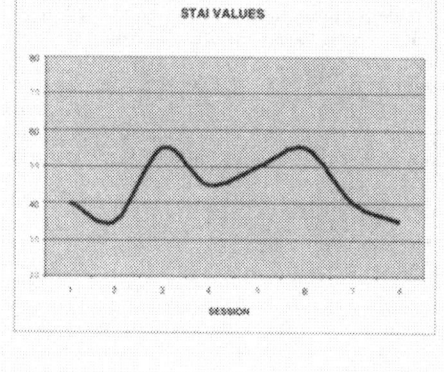

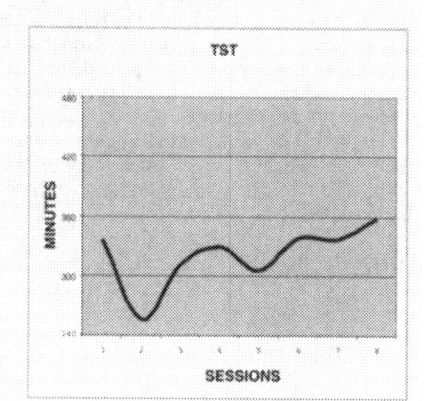

September 29th 2004
Elias Pickwick, MD
25 Nightingale Way
Atlanta, GA

Dear Dr. Pickwick:

Thank you for your referral to our service. I have now had the pleasure of seeing your patient Samuel Busch in the Behavioral Sleep Medicine Service for a total of nine visits between 7/7/04 and 9/22/04. As you know, he is a 62 year old married gentleman with a history of GERD, IBS, and chronic lower back pain who presented with a long standing complaint of trouble initiating and maintaining sleep. This problem became worse about 3 years ago with increasing pressure to perform at work. In 2002 he was let go by his firm. In 2003 his wife was diagnosed with cancer. During this period he gained a substantial amount of weight, and eventually developed a mild sleep apnea. With weight loss, and assistance from you regarding his sleep habits the apnea is now within normal limits, but his sleep pattern continued to be very poor. He was tried on a number of medications with varying degrees of success. Mr. Busch was referred to our service for further assessment.

At our initial work-up, it was felt that Mr. Busch met criteria for Primary Insomnia. Given some of his history, we also considered the possibility that he had either an underlying anxiety disorder, or circadian rhythm disorder, or both. However, it was felt that his frustration about his sleeplessness and poor sleep conditioning needed to be addressed first before we could determine if and how these other factors might be playing a role. Therefore, a Cognitive Behavioral protocol was initiated.

I am very pleased to report that Mr. Busch has done quite well with treatment. The following is a comparison of his average sleep pattern before and after Cognitive Behavioral Therapy:

	BEFORE	AFTER
SL	75 mins.	6.5 mins.
FNA	3.5	0.5
WASO	121 mins.	10 mins.
TST	336	358
SE	63%	95%

As can be seen, Mr. Busch improved in all of the sleep continuity variables we measured. Perhaps of greatest significance is that he achieved this without the use of hypnotic medication. At our last session he was feeling that this amount of sleep was providing adequate energy for him during the day, and he was reporting that he had lost his dread of going to bed at night because he now felt that he had some measure of control. This really seemed like a breakthrough for him.

During the course of treatment, it became clear that Mr. Busch had a tendency to wake early. This was eventually overcome by attenuating the amount of morning light entering his bedroom, and by training him to work out worries and concerns before he went to bed. It should be noted that during our time together, Mr. Busch started a new job as the president of a fledgling company. If anything, this served as an additional stressor to his sleep, but with work he was able to maintain his gains.

At our last visit, relapse prevention strategies were taught. We also suggested that Mr. Busch consider enrolling in a stress-management program and that he might benefit from learning a formal relaxation technique. Both of these things may help him better manage his anxiety and may prevent a recurrence of insomnia. Finally, I made it clear that should he have further problems in the future, he is more than welcome to contact us at that time. In closing, thank you for allowing me to participate in the care of your patient, and if you have any questions regarding his evaluation or treatment here please do not hesitate to contact me.

Austin Doze, Ph.D.
Director, BSMS, Dickens Sleep Center

References

1. Morin CM, Culbert JP, Schwartz SM. Nonpharmacological interventions for insomnia: a meta-analysis of treatment efficacy. Am J Psychiatry 1994; 151(8): 1172–1180.
2. Murtagh DR, Greenwood KM. Identifying effective psychological treatments for insomnia: a meta-analysis. J Consult Clin Psychol 1995; 63(1):79–89.
3. Morin CM, Colecchi C, Stone J, Sood R, Brink D. Behavioral and pharmacological therapies for late-life insomnia: a randomized controlled trial [see comments]. JAMA 1999; 281(11):991–999.
4. Smith MT, Perlis ML, Park A, et al. Comparative meta-analysis of pharmacotherapy and behavior therapy for persistent insomnia. Am J Psychiatry 2002; 159(1):5–11.
5. Edinger JD, Wohlgemuth WK, Radtke RA, Marsh GR, Quillian RE. Cognitive behavioral therapy for treatment of chronic primary insomnia: a randomized controlled trial. JAMA 2001; 285(14):1856–1864.
6. World Health Organization. The ICD-10 Classification of Mental and Behavioural Disorders: Clinical descriptions and diagnostic guidelines. Geneva: World Health Organization, 1992.
7. American Psychological Association. DSM-IV. 4 ed. Washington, D.C.: American Psychiatric Association, 1994.
8. American Sleep Disorders Association. The International Classification of Sleep Disorders: Diagnostic and Coding Manual—Revised. Rochester, MN: American Sleep Disorders Association, 1997.
9. Lichstein KL, Durrence HH, Riedel BW, Taylor DJ, Bush AJ. Epidemiology of sleep: Age, gender, and ethnicity. Mahwah, NJ: Erlbaum, 2002.
10. Perlis ML, Smith MT, Orff HJ, Andrews PJ, Giles DE. Beta/Gamma EEG activity in patients with primary and secondary insomnia and good sleeper controls. Sleep 2001; 24(1):110–117.
11. Merica H, Blois R, Gaillard JM. Spectral characteristics of sleep EEG in chronic insomnia. European Journal of Neuroscience 1998; 10:1826–1834.
12. Merica H, Gaillard JM. The EEG of the sleep onset period in insomnia: a discriminant analysis. Physiol Behav 1992; 52(2):199–204.
13. Freedman R. EEG power in sleep onset insomnia. Electroencephalography and Clinical Neurophysiology 1986; 63:408–413.
14. Lamarche CH, Ogilvie RD. Electrophysiological changes during the sleep onset period of psychophysiological insomniacs, psychiatric insomniacs, and normal sleepers. Sleep 1997; 20(9):724–733.

15. Hall M, Buysse DJ, Nowell PD, et al. Symptoms of stress and depression as correlates of sleep in primary insomnia. Psychosom Med 2000; 62(2):227–230.
16. Perlis ML, Giles DE, Mendelson WB, Bootzin RR, Wyatt JK. Subjective—objective discrepancies in psychophysiologic insomnia: A neurocognitive perspective. J Sleep Res 1997; 6:179–188.
17. Spielman A, Caruso L, Glovinsky P. A behavioral perspective on insomnia treatment. Psychiatr Clin North Am 1987; 10(4):541–553.
18. Bootzin RR. Stimulus control treatment for Insomnia. Proceedings, 80th Annual Convention, APA 1972;395–396.
19. Spielman AJ, Saskin P, Thorpy MJ. Treatment of chronic insomnia by restriction of time in bed. Sleep 1987; 10:45–56.
20. Smith MT, Perlis ML, Giles DE, Pennington JY. Behavioral treatment vs pharmacotherapy for Insomnia—A comparative meta-analyses. American Journal of Psychiatry. 159: 5–11. 2002.
21. Chesson AL, Jr., Anderson WM, Littner M, et al. Practice parameters for the nonpharmacologic treatment of chronic insomnia. An American Academy of Sleep Medicine report. Standards of Practice Committee of the American Academy of Sleep Medicine [In Process Citation]. Sleep 1999; 22(8):1128–1133.
22. Chesson A, Jr., Hartse K, Anderson WM, et al. Practice parameters for the evaluation of chronic insomnia. An American Academy of Sleep Medicine report. Standards of Practice Committee of the American Academy of Sleep Medicine [In Process Citation]. Sleep 2000; 23(2):237–241.
23. Bootzin RR, Epstein D, Ward JM. Stimulus control instructions. In: Hauri P, editor. Case Studies in Insomnia. New York, NY: Plenum Press, 1991: 19–28.
24. Morin CM. Insomnia: Psychological Assessment and Management. New York, NY: Guilford Press, 1993.
25. Shoham-Salomon V, Rosenthal R. Paradoxical interventions: A meta-analysis. J Consult Clin Psychol 1987; 55:22–28.
26. Harvey AG, Payne S. The management of unwanted pre-sleep thoughts in insomnia: distraction with imagery versus general distraction. Behav Res Ther 2002; 40(3):267–277.
27. Buysse DJ, Perlis ML. The evaluation and treatment of insomnia. Journal of Prac Psych and Behav Health 1996; March:80–93.
28. Lichstein KL, Riedel BW, Wilson NM, Lester KW, Aguillard RN. Relaxation and sleep compression for late-life insomnia: a placebo- controlled trial. J Consult Clin Psychol 2001; 69(2):227–239.
29. Haynes SN, Woodward S, Moran R, Alexander D. Relaxation treatment of insomnia. Behavior Therapy 1974; 5:555–558.
30. Freedman R, Papsdorf JD. Biofeedback and progressive relaxation treatment of sleep-onset insomnia: a controlled, all-night investigation. Biofeedback & Self Regulation 1976; 1(3):253–271.
31. Bootzin RR. Evaluation of stimulus control instructions, progressive relaxation, and sleep hygiene as treatments for insomnia. In: Koella WP, Ruther E, Schulz H, editors. Sleep. Stuttgart, Germany: Gustav Fischer Verlag, 1984: 142–144.
32. Borkovec TD, Fowles DC. Controlled investigation of the effects of progressive and hypnotic relaxation on insomnia. J Abnorm Psychol 1973; 82(1):153–158.
33. Wehr TA, Sack DA, Rosenthal NE. Antidepressant effects of sleep deprivation and phototherapy. Acta Psychiatr Belg 1985; 85(5):593–602.

34. Terman M, Schlager DS. Twilight therapeutics, winter depression, melatonin, and sleep. [References]. In: J.M., R.G., editors. Sleep and biological rhythms: Basic mechanisms and applications to psychiatry. New York, NY, US: Oxford University Press, 1990: 113–128.

35. Czeisler CA, Kronauer RE, Mooney JJ, Anderson JL, Allan JS. Biologic rhythm disorders, depression, and phototherapy. A new hypothesis. [Review]. Psychiatr Clin North Am 1987; 10(4):687–709.

36. Chesson AL, Jr., Littner M, Davila D, et al. Practice parameters for the use of light therapy in the treatment of sleep disorders. Standards of Practice Committee, American Academy of Sleep Medicine. Sleep 1999; 22(5):641–660.

37. Cooke KM, Kreydatus MA, Atherton A, Thoman EB. The effects of evening light exposure on the sleep of elderly women expressing sleep complaints. J Behav Med 1998; 21(1):103–114.

38. Sedgwick PM. Disorders of the sleep-wake cycle in adults. Postgrad Med J 1998; 74(869):134–138.

39. Turek FW. Introduction to Chronobiology: Sleep and the Circadian Clock. In: Kryger MH, Roth T, Dement WC, editors. Principles and Practice of Sleep Medicine. Philadelphia, PA: W. B. Saunders Co., 2000: 319–320.

40. Czeisler CA, Khalsa BS. The Human Circadian Timing System and Sleep-Wake Regulation. In: Kryger MH, Roth T, Dement WC, editors. Principles and Practice of Sleep Medicine. Philadelphia, PA: W. B. Mason Co., 2000: 353–376.

41. Turek FW. Introduction: Disorders of Chronobiology. In: Kryger MH, Roth T, Dement WC, editors. Principles and Practice of Sleep Medicine. Philadelphia, PA: W.B. Mason Co., 2000: 589–590.

42. Baker SK, Zee PC. Circadian Disorders of the Sleep-Wake Cycle. In: Kryger MH, Roth T, Dement WC, editors. Principles and Practice of Sleep Medicine. Philadelphia, PA: W.B. Mason Co., 2000: 606–614.

43. Kayumov L, Hawa R, Lowe A, Levin Y, Golbin A, Shapiro CM. Increases in evening- and night-time melatonin levels following brain music therapy for anxiety-associated insomnia. Sleep 2003; 26(Suppl):A99.

44. Bastien CH, Morin CM, Bouchard S et al. Cognitive-Behavioral Treatment of Insomnia: Individual, Group, and Phone Therapy. Sleep 1999; 22(Suppl.): C250.K3.

45. Lichstein KL, Durrence HH, Bayen UJ, Riedel BW. Primary versus secondary insomnia in older adults: subjective sleep and daytime functioning. Psychol Aging 2001; 16(2):264–271.

46. McCrae CS, Lichstein KL. Secondary insomnia: diagnostic challenges and intervention opportunities. Sleep Med Rev 2001; 5(1):47–61.

47. Lichstein KL, Durrence HH, Bayen UJ, Riedel BW. Primary versus secondary insomnia in older adults: subjective sleep and daytime functioning. Psychol Aging 2001; 16(2):264–271.

48. Lichstein KL, Wilson NM, Johnson CT. Psychological treatment of secondary insomnia. 2000. Ref Type: Unpublished Work

49. Perlis ML, Sharpe M, Smith MT, Greenblatt D, Giles D. Behavioral treatment of insomnia: treatment outcome and the relevance of medical and psychiatric morbidity. J Behav Med 2001; 24(3):281–296.

50. Dashevsky BA, Kramer M. Behavioral treatment of chronic insomnia in psychiatrically ill patients. J Clin Psychiatry 1998; 59(12):693–699.

51. Morin CM, Kowatch RA, Wade JB. Behavioral management of sleep distur-
    bances secondary to chronic pain. Journal of Behavior Therapy & Experimen-
    tal Psychiatry 1989; 20(4):295–302.
52. Currie SR, Wilson KG, Pontefract AJ, deLaplante L. Cognitive-behavioral treat-
    ment of insomnia secondary to chronic pain. J Consult Clin Psychol 2000;
    68(3):407–416.
53. Savard J, Morin CM. Insomnia in the context of cancer: a review of a neglected
    problem. J Clin Oncol 2001; 19(3):895–908.
54. Savard J, Simard S, Blanchet J, Ivers H, Morin CM. Prevalence, clinical charac-
    teristics, and risk factors for insomnia in the context of breast cancer. Sleep 2001;
    24(5):583–590.
55. Perlis ML, Giles DE, Mendelson WB, Bootzin RR, Wyatt JK. Psychophysio-
    logical insomnia: the behavioural model and a neurocognitive perspective. J
    Sleep Res 1997; 6:179–188.
56. Perlis ML, Merica H, Smith MT, Giles DE. Beta EEG in insomnia. Sleep Med-
    icine Reviews 2001; 5(5):365–376.
57. Perlis ML, Smith MT, Orff HJ, Enright T, Nowakowski S, Jungquist C, Plotkin
    K. The Effects of Modafinil and CBT on Sleep Continuity in Patients with
    Primary Insomnia. Sleep 2004; 27(4):715–725.
58. Lichstein KL, Peterson BA, Riedel BW, Means MK, Epperson MT, Aguillard
    RN. Relaxation to assist sleep medication withdrawal. Behav Modif 1999;
    23(3):379–402.
59. Tabloski PA, Cooke KM, Thoman EB. A procedure for withdrawal of sleep med-
    ication in elderly women who have been long-term users. J Gerontol Nurs 1998;
    24(9):20–28.
60. Wright Jr KP, Hughes RJ, Kronauer RE, Dijk DJ, Czeisler CA. Intrinsic near-
    24-hour pacemaker period determines limits of circadian entrainmant to a weak
    synchronizer in humans. Proc Natl Aca Sci USA 2001; 98(24):14027–14032.
61. Boivin DB, Duffy JF, Kronauer RE, Czeisler CA. Dose-response relationships
    for resetting of human circadian clock by light. Nature 1996; Feb 8; 379(6565):
    540–542.
62. Boivin DB, Duffy JF, Kronauer RE, Czeisler CA. Sensitivity of the human
    circadian pacemaker to moderately bright light. J Biol Rhythms 1994;
    9(3–4):315–331.
63. Riedel BW, Lichstein KL. Strategies for evaluating adherence to sleep restric-
    tion treatment for insomnia. Behav Res & Therapy 2001; 39:201–212.
64. Borkovec T, Grayson J, O'Brien G, Weerts T. Relaxation treatment of pseudoin-
    somnia and isopathic insomnia: an encephalographic evaluation. Journal of
    Applied Behavioral Analysis 1979; 12:37–54.
65. Lack LC, Bootzin RR. Circadian Rhythm Factors in Insomnia and Their Treat-
    ment. In: Perlis ML, Lichstein KL, editors. Treating Sleep Disorders: Principles
    and Practice of Behavioral Sleep Medicine. Hoboken, NJ: John Wiley and Sons,
    Inc., 2003: 305–343.
66. Beck AT, Rush AJ, Shaw BF, Emery G. Cognitive Therapy of Depression. New
    York: Guilford Press, 1979.
67. Barlow DH, CMG, Cerny JA, KJS. Behavioral treatment of panic disorder.
    Behavior Therapy 1989; 20(2).
68. Perlis M, Aloia M, Millikan A et al. Behavioral treatment of insomnia: A clini-
    cal case series study. J Behav Med 2000; 23(2):149–161.

69. Dobson KS. A meta-analysis of the efficacy of cognitive therapy for depression. J Consult Clin Psychol 1989; 57(3):414–419.

70. Albano AM, Marten PA, Holt CS, Heimberg RG, Barlow DH. Cognitive-behavioral group treatment for social phobia in adolescents. A preliminary study. J Nerv Ment Dis 1995; 183(10):649–656.

71. Barlow DH. Cognitive-behavioral approaches to panic disorder and social phobia. Bull Menninger Clin 1992; 52(2 Suppl A):A14–A28.

72. Harvey L, Inglis SJ, Espie CA. Insomniacs' reported use of CBT components and relationship to long-term clinical outcome. Behav Res Ther 2002; 40(1): 75–83.

73. Backhaus J, Hohagen F, Voderholzer U, Reimann D. Long-term effectiveness of a short-term cognitive-behavioral group treatment for primary insomnia. Eur Arch Psychiatry Clin Neurosci 2001; 251(1):35–41.

74. Bastien CH, Fortier-Brochu E, Rioux I, LeBlanc M, Dayley M, Morin CM. Cognitive Performance and Sleep Quality in the Elderly Suffering From Chronic Insomnia Relationship Between Objective and Subjective Measures. J Psychosom Res 2003;(54):39–49.

75. Qin YL, McNaughton BL, Skaggs WE, Barnes CA. Memory reprocessing in corticocortical and hippocampocortical neuronal ensembles. Philosophical transactions of the royal society of London. Biological Sciences 1997; 352(13).

76. Winson J. Brain and Psyche: The Biology of the Unconscious. New York, NY: Doubleday and Company, 1985.

77. Winson J. The biology and function of REM sleep. Current Opinion in Neurobiology 1999; 3:1–6.

78. Plihal W, Born J. Memory consolidation in human sleep depends on inhibition of glucocorticoid release. Neuroreport 1999; 10(13):2741–2747.

79. Kramer M, Roth T. The mood regulating function of sleep. 1st Europ Congr Sleep Res 1972;563–571.

80. Cartwright RD, Luten A, Young M, Mercer P, Bears M. Role of REM sleep and dream affect in overnight mood regulation: a study of normal volunteers. Psychiatric Research 1998; 81(1):1–8.

81. Perlis ML, Nielsen TA. Mood Regulation, Dreaming and Nightmares: Evaluation of a Desensitization Function of REM Sleep. Dreaming 1993; 3(4):243–257.

82. Adam K, Oswald I. Sleep is for tissue restoration. J R Coll Physicians Lond 1977; 11:376–388.

83. Ebert D, Kaschka WP, Schrell U. Human growth hormone before and after sleep deprivation. European Psychiatry 1992; 7(4):197.

84. Ambrosini PJ, Metz C, Bianchi MD, Rabinovich H, Undie A. Concurrent validity and psychometric properties of the Beck Depression Inventory in outpatient adolescents. J Am Acad Child Adolesc Psychiatry 1991; 30(1):51–57.

85. Bumberry W, Oliver JM, McClure JN. Validation of the Beck Depression Inventory in a university population using psychiatric estimate as the criterion. J Consult Clin Psychol 1978; 46(1):150–155.

86. Robinson BE, Kelley L. Concurrent validity of the Beck Depression Inventory as a measure of depression. Psychol Rep 1996; 79(3 Pt 1):929–930.

87. Schotte CK, Maes M, Cluydts R, De Doncker D, Cosyns P. Construct validity of the Beck Depression Inventory in a depressive population. J Affect Disord 1997; 46(2):115–125.

88. de Beurs E, Wilson KA, Chambless DL, Goldstein AJ, Feske U. Convergent and divergent validity of the Beck Anxiety Inventory for patients with panic disorder and agoraphobia. Depression & Anxiety 1997; 6(4):140–146.

89. Osman A, Kopper BA, Barrios FX, Osman JR, Wade T. The Beck Anxiety Inventory: reexamination of factor structure and psychometric properties. J Clin Psychol 1997; 53(1):7–14.

90. Ware JE, Jr., Sherbourne CD. The MOS 36-item short-form health survey (SF-36). I. Conceptual framework and item selection. Med Care 1992; 30(6):473–483.

91. McHorney CA, Ware JE, Jr., Raczek AE. The MOS 36-Item Short-Form Health Survey (SF-36): II. Psychometric and clinical tests of validity in measuring physical and mental health constructs. Med Care 1993; 31(3):247–263.

92. Brazier JE, Harper R, Jones NM et al. Validating the SF-36 health survey questionnaire: new outcome measure for primary care. BMJ 1992; 305(6846): 160–164.

93. Kerns RD, Turk DC, Rudy TE. The West Haven-Yale Multidimensional Pain Inventory (WHYMPI). Pain 1985; 23(4):345–356.

94. Turk DC, Rudy TE. Toward an empirically derived taxonomy of chronic pain patients: integration of psychological assessment data.

95. Buysse DJ, Reynolds CF, Monk TH, Berman SR, Kupfer DJ. The Pittsburgh Sleep Quality Index: a new instrument for psychiatric practice and research. Psychiatry Res 1989; 28(2):193–213.

96. Bastien C, Vallieres, Morin CM. Validation of the Insomnia Severity Index as an outcome measure for Insomnia research. Sleep Medicine 2001; 2:297–307.

97. Johns MW. Sleepiness in different situations measured by the Epworth Sleepiness Scale. Sleep 1994; 17(8):703–710.

98. Smets EM, Garssen B, Bonke B, De Haes JC. The Multidimensional Fatigue Inventory (MFI) psychometric qualities of an instrument to assess fatigue. J Psychosom Res 1995; 39(3):315–325.

Glossary

A

Actigraph A biomedical instrument, which resembles a wrist watch, that is used to measure and record movement activity.

Actigraphy Algorithms that are applied to movement activity data that allow for the formulation of sleep continuity estimates and/or the quantification activity over a 24-hour day. This method provides an "objective" measure of sleep and may assist with the identification of circadian rhythm disturbances and/or sleep state misperception.

Advanced Sleep Phase Syndrome (ASPS) This Circadian Rhythm Disorder is thought to occur in association with the misalignment between clock time/societal norms and the individual's biologically preferred sleep phase (endogenous rhythm), the notion being that there is an advance such that the individual's internal clock (which regulates preferred sleep phase) is several hours earlier than clock time. Individuals with this disorder often experience irresistible sleepiness in the late afternoon or early evening and thus retire early and then subsequently experience early morning awakenings. A typical sleep schedule for such an individual might be from 8 PM–4 AM. When the individual sleeps within their preferred sleep phase, his/her sleep is normal (i.e., no sleep continuity or architecture disturbance).

Alpha Sleep Typically, the human sleep EEG for NREM sleep is comprised of slow EEG frequencies in the Delta (0.5 Hz–2.0 Hz) and Theta (2.0 Hz–8.0 Hz) ranges. Alpha frequencies (8 Hz–12 Hz) usually signify relaxed wakefulness or arousals from sleep. In subjects with alpha sleep, alpha activity occurs during what is otherwise clear NREM sleep such that that alpha activity is intermingled with Delta and Theta activity. When first observed Alpha (i.e., Alpha–Delta activity) was considered a pathologic form of sleep EEG that was observed in patients with Depression and/or Fibromyalgia. Whether alpha sleep represents a normal variant or pathology is currently a matter of debate.

Autogenic Training This is one of several relaxation techniques. This form of relaxation requires the individual to systematically focus their attention on various regions of the body and to imagine that the region feels warm and/or heavy. The technique is thought to alter blood flow and a way that corresponds to increased parasympathetic and decreased sympathetic activity. The procedure may also have some utility because of its capacity to derail worry and rumination.

B

Beck Anxiety Inventory (BAI)   A self-report instrument designed to measure the severity of anxiety symptoms. This measure is heavily weighted towards physiologic anxiety symptoms (heart palpitations, shortness of breath, etc.) as they might be expressed in panic disorder.

Beck Depression Inventory (BDI)   A self-report instrument designed to measure the severity of depressive symptoms. This measure is heavily weighted towards the cognitive–affective spectrum of the disorder (e.g., dysphoria, depressive cognitions).

Benzodiazepines   Chemically similar substances that bind within the benzodiazepine receptor complex and are thought to promote neuronal hyperpolarization. These substances are used clinically for a broad range of indications including sedation, sleep induction, anxiolysis, myorelaxation, as a treatment for seizures, etc.

Benzodiazepine Receptor Agonists (BZRAs)   BRZAs include substances that are chemically distinct from traditional benzodiazepines but nevertheless bind within the benzodiazepine receptor complex and produce similar effects. Examples include zolpidem (Ambien), zaleplon (Sonata), and s-zopiclone (Estorra).

Beta EEG Activity   A form of high-frequency EEG Activity which is associated with arousal from sleep, and is thought to be correlated with perceived sleep quality and the occurrence of sleep state misperception. The frequency range is from 15 Hz–35 Hz with voltages generally less than 5 microvolts peak to peak. Most investigators allow for this frequency domain to be assessed as two separate bands—Beta-1 (~15 Hz–25 Hz) and Beta-2 (~25 Hz–35 Hz).

Bright Light Therapy   *See* Phototherapy

C

Chronic Insomnia   Insomnia is characterized as chronic when symptoms persist unabated for at least one month, and more typically, for six months or longer. These cutoffs are relatively arbitrary and correspond to traditional medical definitions of what constitutes short and long periods of time.

Circadian Dysrhythmia   Any abnormalities that appear to be related to amplitude or phase distortions in biological or behavioral phenomena that exhibit circadian rhythmicity.

Circadian Pacemaker   The neurobiologic mechanism that is thought to be the "internal clock" responsible for pacing biological or behavioral phenomena over the course of a 24-hour day.

Circadian Rhythm   Biological or behavioral functions that systematically vary over the course of a 24-hour day which may be entrained to light/dark cycles and/or sleep/wakefulness.

Cognitive Restructuring   A therapeutic technique that involves identifying maladaptive cognitions and beliefs, which tend to be automatic, and enables the patient to critically evaluate these thought processes.

Compensatory Strategies Activities or behaviors that individuals engage in that are intended to ameliorate symptoms. While compensatory strategies are intended to provide relief, they often have the effect of perpetuating the acute illness.

D

Delayed Sleep Phase Syndrome (DSPS) This Circadian Rhythm Disorder is thought to occur in association with the misalignment between clock time/societal norms and the individual's biologically preferred sleep phase (endogenous rhythm). The idea is that there is a delay so that the individual's internal clock (which regulates preferred sleep phase) is several hours later than clock time. Individuals with this disorder often do not experience sleepiness until several hours later than what would be convenient given a traditional 9 to 5 work/class schedule. These individuals have difficulty initiating sleep before their biologically preferred sleep phase and have difficulty awakening from sleep when it occurs in the middle of their preferred sleep phase. A typical sleep schedule for such an individual might be from 4 AM to 12 PM. When the individual sleeps within their preferred sleep phase, his/her sleep is normal (i.e., no sleep continuity or architecture disturbance).

Disorders of Initiating and Maintaining Sleep (DIMS) This classification term was used within the original International Classification of Sleep Disorders (ICSD) nosology to describe the class of sleep disorders which had as their chief complaint problems falling and staying asleep.

Downward Titration The systematic reduction of a dose toward an optimal effect. A behavioral sleep medicine example would be in the course of sleep compression therapy, decreasing total sleep opportunity systematically over the 5-week interval.

E

Early Insomnia *See* Initial Insomnia

Early Morning Awakening *See* Terminal Insomnia

Electroencephalography (EEG) A procedure for recording the electrical activity of the brain by means of electrodes placed on the surface of the scalp. These data, in combination with electromyography and electro-occulography, allow for the recording of polysomnograms. The last of these procedures allows for the assessment of the five states which comprise sleep (Stage 1–Stage 4 and REM sleep).

Electromyography (EMG) A procedure for recording the electrical activity of muscle tissue relative to degree of contraction.

Electro-occulography (EOG) A procedure for recording the electrical activity that radiates from the retina. It increases and decreases in voltage as the ocular globe moves toward and away from the EOG electrode.

Epworth Sleepiness Scale (ESS) A self-report instrument designed to measure sleepiness. The ESS requires that the individual rate the likelihood of falling asleep at inappropriate times and places. The time frame over which ratings are to be made is 2 to 4 weeks.

Excessive Daytime Somnolence (EDS) Refers to either the subjective or objective problem of maintaining alertness such that the individual is prone to fall asleep at inappropriate times and places. Subjective assessments of EDS may range from patients complaints to the use of retrospective instruments such as the ESS or the KSS. Objective measures of EDS may be obtained via one of two procedures: The Multiple Sleep Latency Test or The Maintenance of Wakefulness Test. The report of EDS is perhaps the one sign and symptom that can allow for a high level of sensitivity and specificity with respect to the distinction between sleep disorders classified as DOES versus DIMS.

F

Frequency of Nocturnal Awakenings (FNA) The number of times a person awakens during the night. Note: There is really no standard term for this aspect of sleep continuity disturbance. Another frequently used term is "number of awakenings" (NOA).

G

GABAergic Substances Substances that activate, bind at, or alter the activity within the benzodiazepine receptor complex. Examples of GABAergic substances include benzodiazepines like temazepam and "Nonbenzo-Benzodiazepines" like zolpidem.

Gamma EEG Activity A form of high-frequency EEG activity during which wakefulness is associated with sensory processing, attention, and possibly long-term memory formation. The occurrence of such activity during sleep may, like Beta activity, be associated with arousal from sleep, perceived sleep quality, and the occurrence of sleep state misperception. The frequency range is from 35 Hz–45 Hz with voltages generally less than 5 microvolts peak to peak. Some investigators refer to such activity as "40 Hz."

H

Homeostat (Sleep Homeostat) A neurobiologic structure or circuit that is believed to regulate sleep quality and quantity based on the amount and/or quality of prior wakefulness.

Homeostatic Pressure A build-up in the drive for sleep based upon the prolongation of wakefulness.

Hypnogram A graphic representation of sleep stages as they are distributed over the sleep period. The graph has sleep stage on the ordinate (ordered as Wake, REM, Stage 1, Stage 2, Stage 3, and Stage 4) and time on the abscissa.

Hypnotic A substance that produces sleep (somnogenic).

I

Initial Insomnia Insomnia characterized by difficulty falling asleep at bedtime.

Insomnia Severity Index A brief self-report instrument that allows for the assessment of insomnia severity by taking into account intensity of symptoms, chronicity, and occurrence of daytime dysfunction. The index also allows for the resolution of the presenting complaint in terms of initial, middle, and late Insomnia.

Insufficient Sleep Syndrome   An ICSD diagnosis where the complaint of daytime fatigue/sleepiness is primarily related to a curtailed sleep schedule.

International Classification of Sleep Disorders—Revised (ICSD-R)   One of three classification schemes used to define sleep disorders. The alternative nosologies are the DSM-IV-TR (Diagnostic and Statistical Manual for Mental Disorders) and the ICD (International Classification of Disease Manual).

L

Late Insomnia   This term is used with the Hamilton Rating Scale for Depression and is synonymous with Terminal Insomnia and/or early morning awakening.

M

Melatonin   A hormone derived from serotonin and secreted by the pineal gland, particularly in response to darkness. It is thought that this hormone may be important for the regulation of stable sleep-wake cycling.

Middle Insomnia   Insomnia characterized by frequent and/or prolonged awakening(s) in the middle of the night. To be distinguished from initial and late insomnia.

Mixed Insomnia   Insomnia involving any combination of sleep onset, middle of the night, and early morning awakenings.

Multicomponent approach   Interventions that are comprised of more than one form of therapy. With respect to CBT-I, this usually includes at least three components: Stimulus Control Therapy, Sleep Restriction Therapy, and Sleep Hygiene Education.

Multidimensional Pain Inventory (MPI)   A self-report instrument that measures various aspects of the chronic pain experience, including, but not limited to, pain severity, pain-related interference in daily functioning, affective distress, activity level, etc.

Multifactorial Fatigue Inventory (MFI)   A self-report instrument that measures fatigue along several dimensions including mental, physical, etc.

N

NREM Sleep   Literally denotes "Not REM sleep" and refers to Stage 1–Stage 4 sleep.

Narcolepsy   A genetically based syndrome in which patients experience some or all of the following symptoms: EDS and hypnapompic/hypnagogic hallucinations, cateplexy, sleep attacks, and sleep paralysis. The disorder is thought to be a state disassociation disorder characterized by abnormal intrusions of REM into wakefulness.

Neurofeedback   A class of treatments that involve EEG biofeedback or EEG pacing/entrainment to produce EEG sleep (increased Delta/Theta activity).

Nocturnal Myoclonus   *See* Periodic Limb Movement of Sleep

Nonrestorative Sleep   The complaint that sleep quality is poor and the patient feels unrefreshed after a night's sleep. This complaint may occur without concomitant sleep continuity disturbance.

O

Obstructive Sleep Apnea (OSA)   Cessation of airflow during sleep that persists for 10 or more seconds. The apenic event occurs in association with upper airway obstruction. The primary symptoms of OSA include EDS, loud snoring, morning headache and dry mouth, awakenings that occur with the sensation of dyspnea, abnormal motor activity during sleep, etc.

Occult Sleep Disorders   Sleep disorders that exist in the absence of definitive signs and symptoms for the disorder.

P

Paradoxical Insomnia   See Sleep State Misperception.

Parasomnias   Movements and behaviors occurring during sleep. The two broad categories for parasomnias are those that occur during REM and those that occur during NREM, and/or during transitions from NREM sleep. NREM parasomnias include, for example, sleepwalking, sleep talking, sleep terrors, and confusional arousals. REM parasomnias include, for example, nightmares, REM Behavior Disorder (RBD), etc. Parasomnias may or may not associated with sleep continuity disturbance.

Periodic Limb Movements of Sleep (PLMS)   Rapid partial flexion of the foot at the ankle, extension of the big toe, and partial flexion of the knee and hip that occurs during sleep. The movements occur within a periodicity of 20 seconds–60 seconds in a stereotyped pattern lasting 0.5 seconds–5.0 seconds.

Perpetuating Factors   Within the context of the Behavioral Model of Insomnia (i.e., the three-factor model or the Spielman Model) perpetuating factors refer to the behaviors that serve to maintain insomnia as a chronic disorder; behaviors include, but are not limited to, extending sleep opportunity and staying in bed while awake.

Phase Advance   *See* Advanced Sleep Phase Syndrome.

Phase Delay   *See* Delayed Sleep Phase Syndrome.

Phototherapy   The use of high-intensity, full-spectrum light to promote phase shifts in individuals with circadian rhythm disorders. Phototherapy may also be useful in the treatment of Primary Insomnia to promote wakefulness, treat subclinical phase disturbance, and to enhance mood.

Pittsburgh Sleep Quality Index (PSQI)   A self-report instrument that measures various aspects of sleep disturbance. Several domains are assessed including overall degree of sleep disturbance, sleep continuity disturbance, daytime dysfunction, etc.

Poikilothermia   Is a synonym for "cold blooded" (i.e., temperature regulation that is driven by, and determined by, environmental factors).

Polysomnography (PSG)   A procedure for measuring and recording sleep by means of electrodes placed on the surface of the scalp, around the eyes, and on

the orofacial musculature. These data, in combination, allow for the detection and assessment of the five states which comprise sleep (Stage 1–Stage 4 and REM sleep). Additional electrophysiologic measures are acquired to resolve other sleep related phenomena such as OSA and PLMs.

Polysomnogram   A digital or paper recording using PSG techniques of the sleep of an individual.

Precipitating Factors   Within the context of the Behavioral Model of Insomnia precipitating factors refer to the intrinsic and extrinsic stressors that serve to initiate acute bouts of insomnia. The stressors are thought to span the entire biopsychosocial spectrum and include medical illness, life events, etc.

Predisposing Factors   Within the context of the Behavioral Model of Insomnia predisposing factors refer to stable characteristics of the individual that may make him/her prone to acute episodes of insomnia. The traits are thought to span the entire biopsychosocial spectrum and include hyperarousal and hyperactivity, worry and rumination, etc.

Primary Insomnia   The term used within the DSM for chronic insomnia. This classification system also allows for "secondary insomnia." The latter refers to acute or chronic insomnia that is thought be precipitated and perpetuated by a unstable or persistent medical or psychiatric condition.

Prescribed Time In Bed (PTIB)   The clock time that the patient goes to bed each night which is set by the therapist during treatment.

Prescribed Time Out of Bed (PTOB)   The clock time that the patient gets out of bed each morning which is set by the therapist during treatment.

Presleep Arousal Scale   A self-report instrument that measures the severity of somatic and cognitive symptoms experienced while attempting to fall asleep. Symptoms comprising the somatic subscale include feeling hot, tachycardia, physical tension, etc. Symptoms comprising the cognitive subscale include racing thoughts, worries, intrusive thoughts, etc.

Progressive Muscle Relaxation (PMR)   A behavioral intervention designed to teach individuals how to recognize and reduce muscle tension. The procedure involves a series of exercises that consist of systematically tensing and then releasing each of several major skeletal muscle groups. Individuals are instructed to focus attention on the physical sensations of tension and relaxation experienced during these exercises. PMR is often incorporated into multicomponent treatment approaches and may be particularly useful for patients with chronic pain conditions.

Psychophysiological Insomnia   This is the ICSD classification for "primary insomnia." It allows for insomnia to be an independent disease entity and emphasizes the notion that both psychological/behavioral and physiologic factors contribute to the expression illness.

R
Relaxation Training   A set of cognitive/behavioral techniques that diminish physiologic and/or cognitive arousal. The common forms of this intervention are progressive muscle relaxation, diaphragmatic breathing, and autogenic training.

REM Sleep   One of five stages of sleep that may be defined with PSG. This stage is characterized by a fast frequency low voltage EEG (desynchronized EEG) and concomitant rapid eye movements and muscle atonia. REM sleep comprises between 15% and 25% of total sleep time in adults. REM sleep is also referred to as *paradoxical sleep*.

Restless Legs Syndrome (RLS)   A parathesia that occurs in the extremities during the latter half of the day and in association with immobility. Patients describe the sensation as feeling like "pins and needles," "an internal itch," or "a creeping or crawling sensation." These sensation are generally relieved by walking, flexing and/or stretching. RLS may be associated with difficulty initiating sleep and is highly correlated with the occurrence of PLMs.

S

Secondary Insomnia   Insomnia that is thought to be precipitated and perpetuated by medical and/or psychiatric illness.

Sedatives   Within the context of sleep medicine, refers to sleep-inducing or sleep-promoting agents.

SF-36 Health Survey   A self-report instrument that measures "quality of life" in terms of eight factors, including physical and social functioning, role limitations due to physical problems, role limitations due to emotional problems, mental health, energy/vitality, pain and general health perception.

Sigma Activity   This form of EEG activity has a characteristic frequency of 12 Hz–14 Hz. In the normal individual EEG sigma occurs primarily in the form of sleep spindles (a waxing-waning formation that last for 5 seconds–2 seconds). This EEG feature, along with K complexes, defines Stage 2 sleep. Trains of sigma activity that occur without a morphology and for durations of time longer than 2 seconds often occur with the use of benzodiazepine receptor agonists.

Sleep Architecture   Refers to the composition of sleep in terms of PSG stages. Typical sleep architecture variables include percent and minutes of Stage 1–4 and REM sleep.

Sleep Compression   A behavioral technique to increase sleep efficiency whereby Time In Bed is restricted to average total sleep time. Unlike sleep restriction, this technique gradually downwardly titrates TIB over the course of five weeks.

Sleep Continuity   The speed with which sleep is initiated and the degree to which sleep is consolidated. The five variables used to define sleep continuity are Sleep Latency (SL), Frequency of Nocturnal Awakenings (FNA), Wake After Sleep Onset (WASO) time, Total Sleep Time (TST), and Sleep Efficiency (SE%).

Sleep Diary   A means of obtaining prospectively measured sleep continuity and sleep quality. Accomplished by recording on a daily basis the Time to Bed, Time out of Bed, Sleep Latency (SL), Frequency of Nocturnal Awakenings (FNA), Wake After Sleep Onset (WASO) time, Total Sleep Time (TST) and Sleep Efficiency (SE%). Sleep diaries may also contain a variety of other measures that the clinician may wish to sample daily including medication use, alcohol use, etc.

Sleep Efficiency   The ratio of total sleep time to time in bed, multiplied by 100. This variable is often used as the best single measure of sleep continuity.

Sleep Hygiene   A broad set of instructions which recommend and discourage practices that are thought to promote or interfere with good sleep continuity. Examples of such instructions include regularizing bedtime and arise time, restriction of alcohol and caffeine beverages before bedtime, etc.

Sleep Maintenance Insomnia   Difficulty sustaining sleep following sleep onset. *See* Middle Insomnia and/or Late Insomnia.

Sleep Latency (SL)   The time elapsed from lights out (intent to fall asleep) until sleep onset as measured in minutes by self-report, actigraphy, and/or polysomnography.

Sleep Opportunity   The amount of time the individual allots for sleep.

Sleep Pressure   *See* Homeostatic Pressure.

Sleep Restriction Therapy (SRT)   A behavioral treatment that seeks to improve sleep continuity by increasing the homeostatic sleep drive though partial sleep deprivation.

Sleep State Misperception (SSM)   A form of insomnia in which the subjective complaint is not corroborated by traditional PSG methods. That is, there is a substantial sleep continuity complaint where the PSG is within normal limits.

Stage 1 Sleep   A stage of NREM sleep that occurs at sleep onset or that follows arousal from sleep Stages 2, 3, 4, or REM. It consists of a relatively low-voltage EEG with mixed frequency, mainly theta and alpha activity of less than 50% of the scoring epoch. It contains EEG vertex waves and slow, rolling eye movements; no sleep spindles, K complexes, or REMs. Stage 1 normally represents 2%–5% of the major sleep episode.

Stage 2 Sleep   A stage of NREM sleep characterized by the presence of sleep spindles and K complexes present in a relatively low-voltage, mixed-frequency EEG background. High-voltage delta waves may comprise up to 20% of stage 2 epochs; usually accounts for 45%–60% of major sleep episode.

Stage 3 Sleep   A stage of NREM sleep defined by between 20% and 50% time containing EEG waves with a frequency between $0.5\,Hz$ and $2\,Hz$ where each wave peaks at greater than $75\,\mu V$.

Stage 4 Sleep   A stage of NREM sleep defined by between 50% and 100% time containing EEG waves with a frequency between $0.5\,Hz$ and $2\,Hz$ where each wave peaks at greater than $75\,\mu V$.

State Trait Anxiety Inventory (STAI)   A self-report instrument that measures anxiety along one of two dimensions (State versus Trait). This instrument appears to be more sensitive to general anxiety (vs panic disorder).

Stimulus Control Therapy (SCT)   A behavioral therapy for insomnia that attempts to limit the number of associations that exist for sleep related stimuli.

T

Terminal Insomnia   A type of insomnia in which the patient's major complaint is early morning awakening.

Time to Bed (TTB)   The average time, for some interval, that the individual retires to bed with the intention of going to sleep. This parameter is usually calculated from 1–2 weeks worth of sleep diary data.

Time Out of Bed (TOB)   The clock time a person gets out of bed in the morning.

Total Sleep Time (TST)   The amount of actual sleep time for a given sleep opportunity period. May be estimated without calculation by the individual, derived from sleep diary data, calculated from actigraphy or represent the sum of PSG measured sleep stages. On sleep diaries, TST may be calculated as follows: Sleep Opportunity – (SL + WASO).

U

Upward Titration   The systematic increase of a dose towards an optimal effect. A behavioral sleep medicine example would be in the course of sleep restriction therapy, increasing sleep opportunity systematically based criterion values for sleep efficiency.

W

Wake After Sleep Onset (WASO)   The amount of wake time for a given sleep opportunity period. May be estimated without calculation by the individual, derived from sleep diary data, calculated from actigraphy or represent the sum of PSG measured wakefulness.

Z

Zaleplon   A short acting (Half life: 0–2.0) BZRA.

Zopiclone (Eszopiclone)   A medium half-life (4.5–7.5)BZRA compound.

Zolpidem   A medium half-life (2.5–5.5) BZRA compound.

Appendices

1
The Calculation of Sleep Efficiency

At first blush, the equation (TST/TIB) seems straightforward and something that requires no further explanation.

$$TST = TIB - (SL + WASO)$$
$$TIB = \text{The difference between PTOB and PTTB}$$

Where PTTB refers to *Prescribed Time To Bed* and PTOB refers to *Prescribed Time Out of Bed*.

In practice the designation of what constitutes "TIB" or the correct denominator in the SE ratio may be challenging. Under the simplest of circumstances, where the patient is compliant with the Prescribed Time To Bed and the Prescribed Time Out of Bed the calculation is indeed straightforward. If the patient is prescribed a midnight to 6 am sleep schedule, then the denominator is 360 minutes. If, however, the patient is non-compliant with the prescribed sleep schedule and phase delays or advances his/her bedtime or waketime, then there is a question about what constitutes TIB as the patient's PTTB or PTOB is not what was prescribed.

Phase Advance of the Prescribed Bedtime. In the case of the phase advance of bedtime, where the patient goes to bed earlier then prescribed (e.g., 11 PM rather than midnight) TIB should be based upon the *actual* PTTB (thus 11–6 or 420 minutes). This said, the decision on how to proceed with titration is no longer simply based on sleep efficiency. If the patient successfully "cheats" (>90% SE is achieved), then upward titration may occur from the new bench mark of 11 PM. If the patient is not successful with his/her attempt to "cheat" (90% SE), then there are two options. First, one could recalculate the PTTB based on the current total sleep time average. For example, if the patient is now averaging 5.5 hours of sleep, then the new time might be set at 12:30–6 AM. Second, one could simply restart SRT with the original prescribed sleep schedule (i.e., 12–6). Which of these options is chosen may be a matter of judgment regarding the patient's resolve, and factors that may have influenced the variability of average total sleep time.

Phase Delay of the Prescribed Bedtime. In the case of the phase delay of bedtime, where the patient goes to bed later then prescribed (e.g., 1 AM rather than midnight), TIB is again based upon the actual PTTB (thus 1–6 or 300 minutes). This said, the decision on how to proceed with titration may again not simply be based on sleep efficiency. In this case, it is likely that the greater than intended phase delay of bedtime will result in sleep efficiencies of greater than 90%. The central issue is how to handle the "noncompliance." In this scenario, it can be argued that the patient is "super" complaint in one respect, but not another; compliant with the treatment

related "priming of the sleep homeostat" but not compliant with sleep scheduling. The more important quandary, however, is "how should one proceed with SRT?" Should treatment continue based on the known effects of the 5-hour window or the original estimate which allowed for a 6-hour window. Our sense is that the former strategy is better—upward titration should now be based on the new benchmark of 1 AM. The patient has already demonstrated that she/he can stay awake to the later hour and that they can sleep efficiently within this context. One note of caution, however, is that some patients may be staying up later, "to get things done." Unless given firm direction, such patients may continue to stay up later out of a sense that they can use the extra time. In our experience, it may be best to insist that these patients go to bed at the originally prescribed time (12–6). This can help demonstrate to them that they can, in fact, fall asleep earlier, and some work may be needed to problem solve other times that can be devoted to whatever activities they feel are not getting done as a result of going to bed earlier.

Phase Advance of the Prescribed Waketime. In the case of the phase advance of waketime, where the patient wakes and gets out of bed earlier then the prescribed time (e.g., 5 AM rather than 6 AM), but where the patient's intent was to sleep until 6 AM, TIB here is based upon the intended PTOB and would still be 6 hours. This is so because the "intent" was to be able to sleep 360 minutes, but this was not achieved. To stick with a literal interpretation of TIB here would produce a sleep efficiency of 100%, which is clearly not a good representation of what occurred. In actuality, the patient woke early and was experiencing terminal insomnia. Titration in this case should proceed solely on the basis of sleep efficiency. On the other hand, if for a particular night or series of nights, the patient sets her/his alarm to wake at 5 AM because she/he needed to do so (intended to do so, e.g., to catch a flight), then TIB would only be 5 hours, because in this case the patient was in fact intent on waking at 5 AM. Sleep efficiency here again might be "artificially" high and the therapist might want to see how the patient does with the intended 12–6 schedule, before proceeding with upward titration.

Phase Delay of the Prescribed Waketime. In the case of the phase delay of waketime, where the patient gets out of bed later then prescribed (e.g., 7 AM rather than 6 AM), TIB is again based upon the actual PTOB (7 hours). As with the Phase Advance of bedtime, this scenario is more complex as the patient may or may not have successfully "cheated." If the patient successfully "cheated" (>90% SE is achieved), then upward titration may occur from the new bench mark of 7 AM. If the patient was not successful with her/his attempt to "cheat" (<90% SE), then there are again two options:—(1) recalculate the PTOB based on the current total sleep time average or (2) restart SRT with the original prescribed sleep schedule.

Calculating TIB with Stimulus Control Instructions. The practice of SCT instruction raises another potential ambiguity regarding the appropriate denominator (TIB) to be used in calculating sleep efficiency. That is, if the patient is compliant with SCT, how is *time out of bed* factored into the calculation of *Time in Bed*? For example, the sleep schedule is set at 12 AM to 6 AM and the patient practices STC appropriately and gets out of bed for 60 minutes over the course of the night. In this instance, the denominator would still be set at 360 minutes even though the patient was not technically in bed for the full 360 minutes. Again this is so because the intent was 360 minutes, but this was not achieved. Thus again, the patient is exhibiting insomnia and to stick with the literal interpretation of TIB here would misrepresent this fact. Titration in this case should be solely based on sleep efficiency.

2
Example of Clinic Brochure: Front and Back

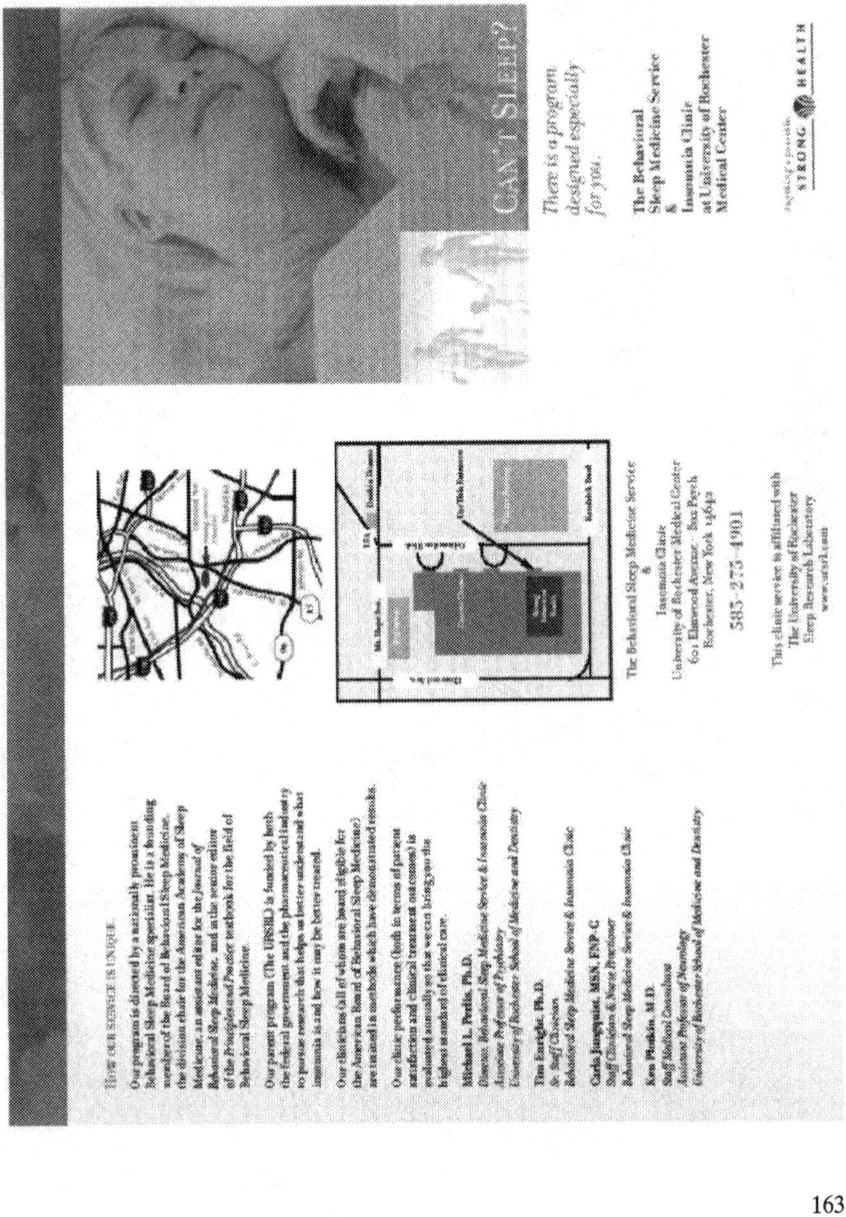

YOU ARE NOT ALONE.

More than one in four people experience insomnia from time to time and sometimes it even will suffer from a chronic form of the disorder. Despite the prevalent belief that insomnia is not a serious problem, there is substantial evidence which shows that untreated and persistent insomnia is associated with:

- Reduced quality of life
- Poor work performance
- increased occurrence of accidents
- Risk for medical illness
- Risk for psychiatric illness

Fortunately, for the 10-20% percent of Americans who suffer from insomnia, there is help. Recent advances in Sleep Medicine enable sleep experts to help the majority of troubled sleepers, often without medication.

WHAT TYPES OF SLEEP PROBLEMS ARE TREATED?

We evaluate and treat patients who have difficulty falling asleep, difficulty staying asleep or difficulty sleeping on a schedule that allows them to function well in their work.

We also specialize in the diagnosis and treatment of sleep disturbances associated with:

- Secondary to chronic pain, cancer, and depression and/or anxiety
- Nightmares and night terrors
- Jet lag

Also available are alternative treatments for patients who have difficulty tolerating CPAP treatment for obstructive sleep apnea.

Although we specialize in adult sleep disorders, children and adolescents may also be seen in the clinic.

WHAT HAPPENS AT THE INSOMNIA CLINIC?

Your sleep evaluation will involve a series of steps. It begins with an initial consultation during which you will be asked to complete a series of questionnaires and to undergo a clinical interview. This information will help us evaluate the factors that affect your sleep and daytime functioning.

Following the assessment, we will review our recommendations with you and your primary care physician or health care provider. Follow-up treatment can be conducted at tour clinic or by your health care provider, depending on the nature of the intervention.

WHAT KIND OF TREATMENT CAN I EXPECT?

For patients with Primary or Secondary Insomnia, the first line of intervention is usually behavioral. Behavioral treatment is based upon the concept that chronic insomnia (greater than 3 weeks) is maintained by a variety of physical and behavioral factors that have little or nothing to do with acute insomnia (one or two days). The factors that maintain the chronic insomnia are the ones targeted for treatment.

Clinical studies have shown that behavioral treatment for insomnia is effective, producing long-lasting results that are comparable to or exceed those of sleeping pills.

For overnight weekly syndrome see results required to get proper good sleep and to help them continue sleeping well. Follow-up recommendations are made to ensure that the results are sustained.

In some cases, a laboratory sleep study may be arranged and/or medications may be recommended. In all cases, we will work closely with your health care provider to ensure that our care is coordinated.

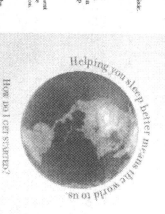

Helping you sleep better means the world to us.

HOW DO I GET STARTED?

Appointments for the
Behavioral Sleep Medicine Service
&
Insomnia Clinic
at URMC may be arranged by calling
585-275-1901

3
Example of Treatment Graphs

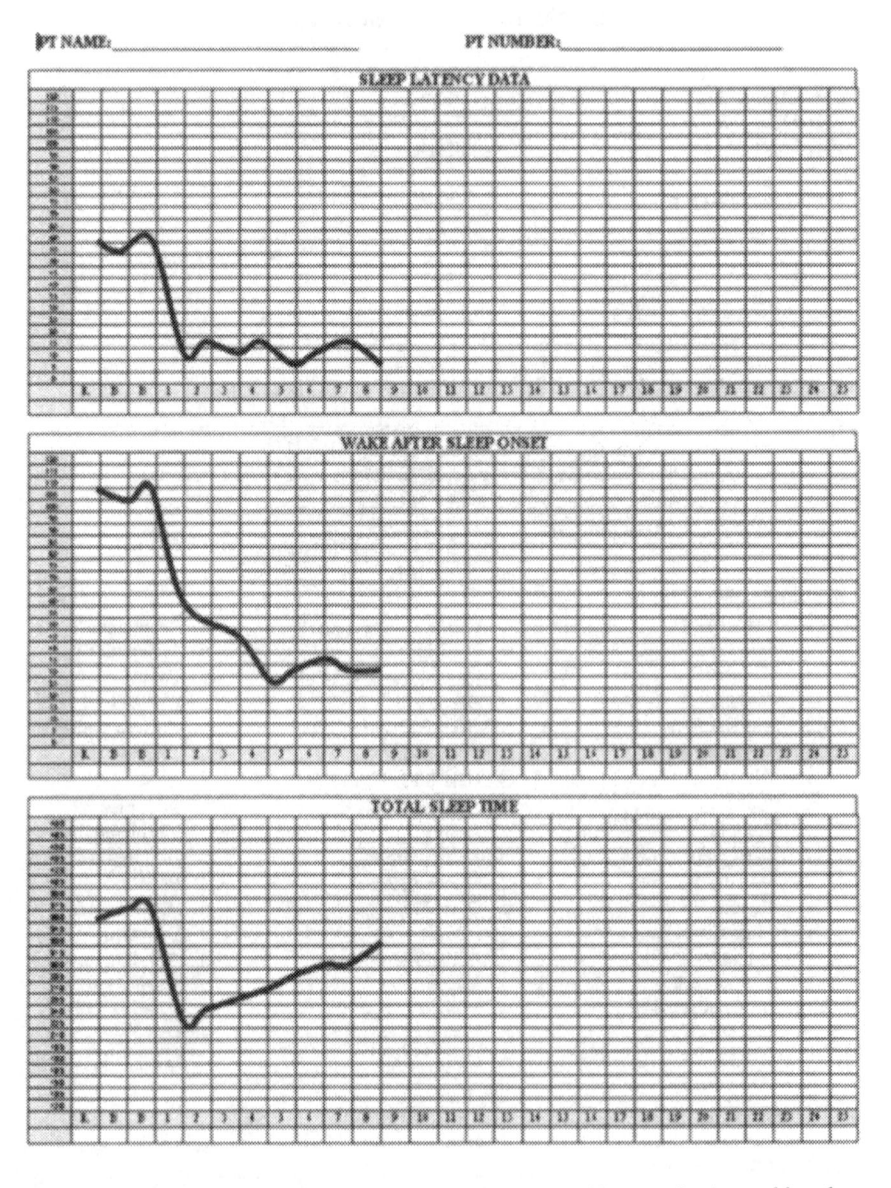

Note   These graphs are completed by hand each week. In this example, the weekly values are not coded along the abscissa. Coding the numeric values allows for easier chart review for the clinics that do end of year program evaluations.

4A
Medical History Checklist

MEDICAL HISTORY INFORMATION FORM

Current weight: _____   Name: _____
Current height: _____   Date: _____
Weight 5 years ago: _____ BMI: _____

List of medications:

Med	Dose	Schedule	Reason taking it

Put checkmark in the box:

- ❑ Head injury
- ❑ Hemorrhage
- ❑ Meningitis
- ❑ Migraine
- ❑ Multiple Sclerosis
- ❑ Parkinson's
- ❑ Seizures
- ❑ Stroke
- ❑ Shingles
- ❑ Chest pain
- ❑ Irregular Heart Rhythm
- ❑ Congestive Heart Failure
- ❑ Heart Attack
- ❑ Vision problems
- ❑ Blood clots
- ❑ Asthma

- ❑ Colitis
- ❑ Constipation
- ❑ Gastric Ulcer Disease
- ❑ Gastric bleeding
- ❑ Pancreatitis
- ❑ Heartburn
- ❑ Esophageal Reflux
- ❑ Cystitis
- ❑ Kidney Stones
- ❑ Menopause
- ❑ Ovarian Cysts
- ❑ Pelvic Inflammatory Disease
- ❑ Kidney failure
- ❑ Blood disorders
- ❑ Chronic Pain

- ❑ Pneumonia
- ❑ Tuberculosis
- ❑ Cancer
- ❑ Diabetes
- ❑ Thyroid problems
- ❑ Obesity
- ❑ Gout
- ❑ Arthritis
- ❑ Fibromyalgia
- ❑ HIV disease
- ❑ Psoriasis
- ❑ Hives or rashes
- ❑ Dental problems
- ❑ Grinding teeth
- ❑ Sleep Apnea
- ❑ Restless Legs
- ❑ Hepatitis
- ❑ Liver Disease

Other: _____

List Surgeries with dates: _____

_____

4B
Medical Symptom Checklist

MEDICAL SYMPTOMS CHECKLIST

Have you had any of the following in the past two weeks: (if you check yes, state number of days and severity)?

Yes	# of Days	Severity Rating (1 low–5 high)
_____ Back pain	_____	_____
_____ Bruising	_____	_____
_____ Chest pain	_____	_____
_____ Cold symptoms	_____	_____
_____ Constipation	_____	_____
_____ Daytime fatigue	_____	_____
_____ Daytime sleepiness	_____	_____
_____ Diarrhea	_____	_____
_____ Difficulty swallowing	_____	_____
_____ Dizziness	_____	_____
_____ Double vision	_____	_____
_____ Eye strain	_____	_____
_____ Fainting spells	_____	_____
_____ Flatulence	_____	_____
_____ Flu symptoms	_____	_____
_____ Flushing	_____	_____
_____ Foot pain	_____	_____
_____ Genital infection	_____	_____
_____ Genital pain	_____	_____
_____ Headaches	_____	_____
_____ Heart palpitations	_____	_____
_____ Heartburn/GERD	_____	_____
_____ Menstrual pain	_____	_____
_____ Muscle pain	_____	_____
_____ Muscular weakness	_____	_____
_____ Neck pain	_____	_____
_____ Numbness	_____	_____
_____ Persistent cough	_____	_____
_____ Ringing in the ears	_____	_____
_____ Shortness of breath	_____	_____
_____ Sore throat	_____	_____
_____ Swelling	_____	_____
_____ Toothaches	_____	_____
_____ Trouble swallowing	_____	_____
_____ Other	_____	_____

4C
The Sleep Disorders Symptom Checklist

THE SDS-CL	NEVER	SELDOM	SOMETIMES	OFTEN	FREQUENTLY
IT TAKES ME 30 OR MORE MINUTES TO FALL ASLEEP					
I WAKE UP FOR 30 OR MORE MINUTES DURING THE NIGHT					
I WAKE UP 30 OR MORE MINUTES PRIOR TO MY ALARM					
I PREFER TO GO TO BED EARLY (BEFORE 10) AND WAKE UP EARLY (BEFORE 5:30)					
I PREFER TO GO TO BED LATE (AFTER 1) AND WAKE UP LATE (AFTER 9AM)					
I AM PRONE TO FALL ASLEEP AT INAPPROPRIATE TIMES OR PLACES					
I WAKE UP WITH HEADACHES IN THE MORNING					
I WAKE UP WITH A DRY MOUTH IN THE MORNING (COTTON MOUTH)					
I SNORE					
MY SNORING IS SO LOUD, THAT MY BEDPARTNER COMPLAINS					
I WAKE UP CHOKING OR GASPING FOR AIR					
MY BEDPARTNER HAS NOTICED THAT I SEEM TO STOP BREATHING					
I GET UNCOMFORTABLE SENSATIONS IN MY LEGS					
IN THE EVENING MY LEGS FEEL "RESTLESS"					

THE SDS-CL	NEVER	SELDOME	SOMETIMES	OFTEN	FREQUENTLY
I OFTEN FEEL THAT I HAVE TO GET UP AND WALK AROUND					
I HAVE BEEN TOLD THAT I AM A RESTLESS SLEEPER					
MY BEDPARTNER COMPLAINS THAT I MOVE AROUND A LOT AT NIGHT					
WHEN EXCITED (E.G., ANGER OR HUMORED) I FEEL PHYSICALLY WEAK					
WHEN I AM FALLING ASLEEP, I EXPERIENCE SCARY DREAM LIKE IMAGES					
WHEN I AM FIRST AWAKENING, I EXPERIENCE SCARY DREAM LIKE IMAGES					
WHEN I AM FIRST AWAKENING, I FEEL LIKE I CAN'T MOVE					
I HAVE NIGHTMARES, PARTICULARLY IN THE FIRST ½ OF THE NIGHT					
I HAVE NIGHTMARES, PARTICULARLY IN THE LATTER ½ OF THE NIGHT					
FOR NO REASON, I AWAKEN SUDDENLY, STARTLED, AND FEELING AFRAID					

4D
Sleep Environment Checklist

SLEEP ENVIRONMENT QUESTIONNAIRE

1. I use an alarm clock five or more days a week.

    True   False   Not Applicable

2. I keep the temperature in the bedroom so cold that I have 2 or more blankets on the bed to stay warm at night.

    True   False   Not Applicable

3. The blinds and curtains in the bedroom are so effective that at sunrise the room is so dark its hard to tell that the sun came up.

    True   False   Not Applicable

4. I have spent real time and money making sure that my mattress and pillow are perfect for me.

    True   False   Not Applicable

5. During the night, my bedroom is insulated so well that I rarely if ever hear outside noise from the road, neighbors, etc.

    True   False   Not Applicable

6. House noise from the radiators, floor boards, etc. is so minimal that I am rarely aware of such sounds.

    True   False   Not Applicable

7. My home is a safe place. My partner and/or pet and/or the locks and alarm system and/or concern and support of my neighbors provide me a level of comfort such that I rarely if ever worry about being safe at night.

    True   False   Not Applicable

8. On three or more nights per week, I engage in two or more of the following behaviors in the bedroom: watch TV, read, plan, worry, work, clean, or eat.

    True   False   Not Applicable

9. My pets rarely, if ever, keep me from falling asleep or wake me up during the night.

    True   False   Not Applicable

10. My bed partner's sleep schedule or habits while in bed (reading, moving about, stealing the covers, snoring, etc.) rarely, if ever, disturb my sleep.

    True   False   Not Applicable

11. My child's/children's sleep schedule or habits while in bed or during the night rarely if ever disturb my sleep.

    True   False   Not Applicable

4E
Motivation for Change Index

MFCI
(Motivation For Change Index)

1. Because of my insomnia I can't (Please list)

_____   _____
_____   _____
_____   _____
_____   _____
_____   _____

2. If there were a treatment we could use that would, as of tomorrow, fix your insomnia—in what way(s) would your life be better?

_____   _____
_____   _____
_____   _____
_____   _____
_____   _____

3. If there were a treatment we could use that would fix your insomnia how many hours per week would you be willing to invest in the process?
_____ 1 hour _____ 2 hour _____ 4 hour _____ 8 hour _____ 10 hour

4. If there were a treatment we could use that would fix your insomnia BUT it would take time, how long would you be willing to wait?
_____ 1 week _____ 2 week _____ 4 week _____ 8 week _____ 10 weeks

5. If there were a treatment we could use that would fix your insomnia BUT to get better it would mean that you'd get worse before you get better, how much worse would you be willing to get?
_____ 10% _____ 20% _____ 40% _____ 80% _____ 100%

6. To make a difference in your life, how much improvement would represent a real accomplishment?
_____ 10% _____ 20% _____ 40% _____ 80% _____ 100%

5
Single Day Sleep Diary

WESTERN PSYCHIATRIC INSTITUTE AND CLINIC SLEEP AND CHRONOBIOLOGY CENTER PITTSBURGH SLEEP DIARY (PghSD)

Please keep this booklet by your bed, and fill it out last thing at night and first thing in the morning. There are 14 sheets in the booklet, one sheet for each night of sleep. Please fill out the left half of the sheet last thing at night, the right half first thing the following morning. We realize that estimates of time to fall asleep and time awake during the night are not going to be exact, just do the best you can.

When answering questions about how well you slept, your alertness, and mood on awakening, please consider the line to represent your own personal range. Place a mark somewhere along the line to represent your feelings at that time. We are using the line so that you are not required to give "yes" or "no" answers, but can give one of a whole range of possible answers. Please try to use the whole scale, rather than simply putting your marks at one end or the other.

NAME _____   ID# ____

SLEEP DIARY   **BEDTIME**   **KEEP BY BED**

Please fill out this part of the diary last thing at night.

day _____   date _____

Today, when did you have: (if none, write "none")

breakfast _____   lunch _____   dinner _____

How many of the following did you have in each time period? *(if none, leave blank)*

	before or with breakfast	after breakfast before/with lunch	after lunch before/with dinner	after dinner
caffeinated drinks	_____	_____	_____	_____
alcoholic drinks	_____	_____	_____	_____
cigarettes	_____	_____	_____	_____
cigars/pipes/plugs (of chewing tobacco)	_____	_____	_____	_____

Which drugs and medications did you take today? *(prescribed & over the counter)*

Name	Time	Dose
_____	_____	_____
_____	_____	_____

What exercise did you take today? (if none, check here) ☐

start _____   end _____   type _____

start _____   end _____   type _____

How many daytime naps did you take today? (if none, write O) _____ *give times for each*:

start _____   end _____   start _____   end _____

172

WESTERN PSYCHIATRIC INSTITUTE AND CLINIC SLEEP AND CHRONOBIOLOGY CENTER PITTSBURGH SLEEP DIARY (PghSD)

SLEEP DIARY   <u>**WAKETIME**</u>   **KEEP BY BED**

Please fill out this part of the diary first thing in the <u>morning</u>.

day _____ date _____

went to bed last night at _____

lights out at _____

minutes until fell asleep _____

finally woke at _____

Awakened by (*check one*):

alarm clock/radio ❏

someone whom I asked to wake me ❏

noises ❏

just woke ❏

After falling asleep, woke up this many times during the night (circle)

    0   1   2   3   4   5 or more

<u>total</u> number of minutes awake _____

- woke to use bathroom (circle # times)
      0   1   2   3   4   5 or more
- awakened by noises/child/bedpartner (circle # times)
      0   1   2   3   4   5 or more
- awakened due to discomfort or physical complaint (circle # times)
      0   1   2   3   4   5 or more
- just woke (circle # times)
      0   1   2   3   4   5 or more

Ratings (place a mark somewhere along the line):

Sleep Quality:

very bad _____ very good

Mood on Final Wakening:

very tense _____ very calm

Alertness on Final Wakening:

very sleepy _____ very alert

6
"Week at a Glance" Sleep Diary

NAME _____

DATE _____

COMPLETE IMMEDIATELY UPON AWAKENING

	MON	TUES	WED	THURS	FRI	SAT	SUN		MEAN
TIME TO BED (CLOCK TIME)									
TIME OUT OF BED (CLOCK TIME)									
TIME TO BED (DEV FRM 11)									
TIME OUT OF BED (DEV FRM 7)									
SL TIME TO FALL ASLEEP (min)									
NOA NUMBER TIMES AWAKENED (#)									
WASO AMOUNT OF TIME AWAKE (min)									
TOB TOTAL TIME OUT OF BED (min)									
TST TOTAL SLEEP TIME (min)									

SE AND TIB TO BE AUTO-CACULATED

COMPLETE IMMEDIATELY PRIOR TO BED
REGARDING HOW YOU FELT TODAY:

	MON	TUES	WED	THUR	FRI	SAT	SUN		MEAN
TYPICAL DAY? (YES/NO)**									
FATIGUE (NONE 0—1—2—3—4—5 ALOT)									
STRESS (NONE 0—1—2—3—4—5 ALOT)									
ALERT (NOT VERY 0—1—2—3—4—5 VERY)									
CONCENTRATION (POOR 0—1—2—3—4—5 GOOD)									
MOOD (BAD 0—1—2—3—4—5 GOOD)									
TIME SPENT EXERCISING (MIN.)									
TIME SPENT OUTSIDE TODAY (MIN.)									
# ALCOHOLIC BEVERAGES									
PRESCRIPTIONS TODAY (YES/NO)									
OTC MEDS TODAY (YES/NO)									
PAIN TODAY (NONE 0—1—2—3—4—5 ALOT)									
HEALTH (FELT FINE 0—1—2—3—4—5 BAD)									
MENSTRUATE TODAY (YES/NO)									
MENSTRUAL PAIN (FELT FINE 0—1—2—3—4—5 BAD)									

**PLEASE INDICATE ON THE BACK OF THIS SHEET WHY ANY GIVEN DAY WAS NOT TYPICAL AND/OR WHAT
MEDICATIONS YOU TOOK ON ANY GIVEN DAY.

Index

A

Actigraphy, 31–33
  advantages of, 31
  device (photo), 32
  functions of, 31
  output report, 32
  in treatment phase, 32
Acute insomnia, versus chronic
    insomnia, 3
Advanced Sleep Phase Syndrome,
    87–88
Alarm clock, use of, 72, 80
Alcohol use, effects on sleep, 39, 76–78
Alpha-Delta sleep, 31
American Academy of Sleep Medicine
    (AASM)
  certification by, 24
  web site for, 24
Antidepressants
  as treatment option, 44, 46
  types of, 45
Anxiety
  anti-anxiety medications, 45
  assessment instrument, 27
  and insomnia, 42
Assessment. *See* Diagnosis of insomnia;
    Sleep assessment
Autogenic training, goal of, 19

B

Bathing, hot bath and sleep, 73
Beck Anxiety Inventory, 27
Beck Depression Inventory (BDI), 27
Bed, excessive time in, 8–9
Bedroom. *See* Sleep environment

Behavioral factors and insomnia,
    38–40
  assessment of, 38–40
  counter fatigue measures, 39
  extending sleep opportunity, 39
  rituals/strategies, 39
  self-medication, 39
Behavioral model of insomnia, 7–11
  conditioned arousal in, 9–10
  four-factor model, 10–11
  patient introduction to, 52–55
  perpetuating factors, 8–10, 52–55
  precipitating factors, 8, 10, 52–53
  predisposing factors, 7–8, 10, 52–53
  stimulus control perspective, 9–11
  stress diathesis model, 7–9
Behavioral Sleep Medicine
    Certification, 24
Benzodiazepines
  listing of types, 45
  side effects, 110
  for sleep state misperception, 87
  as treatment option, 44
Biological factors, in insomnia, 7–8
Bipolar disorder
  and insomnia, 42
  risks and therapy, 14, 16, 20
Breathing, diaphragmatic, 19
Brochure, for clinic, 163–164

C

Caffeine, guidelines for use, 71, 75–76
Catastrophic thinking
  cognitive restructuring for, 89–96
  most common worries, 90

CBTs. *See* Cognitive-behavioral
    therapies
Certification, by American Academy of
    Sleep Medicine (AASM), 24
Chronic insomnia, versus acute
    insomnia, 3
Circadian dysrhythmia, 87–88
    and actigraphy, 31
    treatment of, 87–88
    types of, 31
Circadian regulation, 14*n*
Classical conditioning
    learned sleep-prevention
        associations, 2
    and stimulus control therapy (SCT),
        14
Clinic. *See* Sleep medicine clinic
Clinical assessment. *See* Sleep
    assessment
Clinic chart, 25–26
    purpose of, 25–26
Clinicians. *See* Sleep medicine
    practitioners
Cognition, during sleep, 65–66
Cognitive-behavioral therapies
    case example, 121–141
    client-therapist relationship, 24–25
    clinic chart, 25–26
    clinician office, 25
    clinician training/expertise, 23–24
    cognitive therapy, 17–18
    contraindications for, 41–43
    course of treatment, 21–22
    environment of clinic, 25
    focus of, 9
    indications for, 36–41
    neurofeedback, 21
    patient acceptance, reasons for, 50
    patient appropriateness for, 22–23
    patient assessment. *See* Sleep
        assessment
    patient nonadherence, 64–70
    patient questions/concerns, 105–120
    phototherapy, 19–20
    presenting as treatment option,
        44
    relaxation training, 19
    sleep compression, 20–21
    sleep hygiene education, 17

sleep restriction therapy (SRT),
    14–16
stimulus control therapy (SCT),
    12–14
structuring sessions. *See* Cognitive-
    behavioral therapy sessions
Cognitive-behavioral therapy sessions
    clinician's report, case study, 121–141
    duration of sessions, 21–22
    first patient contact, 33
    intake evaluation, 21, 34–48
    patient concerns/problems, 105–120
    sleep hygiene, 70–82
    sleep titration, 63–70, 83–104
    structuring sessions. *See* Cognitive-
        behavioral therapy sessions
    time required for treatment, 21
    treatment initiation, 49–62
Cognitive restructuring
    as adjunctive mode, 18
    for catastrophic thinking, 89–96
    effectiveness of, 89–90
    for nonadherence, 67
    steps in, 90
Cognitive therapy, 17–18
    cognitive restructuring, 18
    distraction and imagery, 18
    paradoxical intention, 18
Compensatory strategies. *See*
    Behavioral factors and insomnia
Compliance. *See* Patient compliance
Conditioned arousal, 9–10
    evaluation at intake, 41
Contraindications for therapy, 14, 16,
    20, 41–43

D
Daytime fatigue, 5–6
    assessment measure for, 27, 61
    modafinil for, 61–62
    and napping, 80–81
    patient concerns about, 113–115
    patient reports, 38
    and quality of sleep, 5
    and sleep restriction therapy (SRT),
        61–62
    and treatment initiation, 61–62
Delayed Sleep Phase Syndrome,
    87–88

Dementia, and insomnia, 42
Depression
    assessment instrument, 27
    and insomnia, 42
Diagnosis of insomnia
    acute versus chronic insomnia, 3
    daytime fatigue in, 5–6
    duration criteria, 2, 3, 40
    frequency of symptoms, 3–4
    insomnia versus short sleep, 5
    intensity of symptoms, 4–5
    patient descriptions, 7
    subjective criteria in, 5
Diagnostic and Statistical Manual of
    Mental Disorders-IV, on primary
    insomnia, 1, 5
Diaphragmatic breathing, goal of, 19
Diary. See Sleep diary
Disorders of initiation and
    maintenance (DIMS), 36–37
Distraction and imagery, 18

E
Electroencephalogram (EEG)
    and neurofeedback therapy, 21
    NREM disturbances, 5
    and polysomography, 30
    substance abuse indications, 88
Electromyography (EMG), and
    polysomography, 30
Electroocculography (EOG), and
    polysomography, 30
Epilepsy, risk and therapy, 14, 16
Epworth Sleepiness Scale (ESS), 27, 61
Excessive Daytime Sleepiness 6, 61
Exercise, effects on sleep, 39, 73–74
Eye conditions, risks and therapy, 20

F
Falls, risks and therapy, 14, 16
Fatigue during day. See Daytime
    fatigue
Fluid intake, reducing, 75
Forcing sleep, impossibility of, 79–80
Four-factor model, 10–11
Free running rhythms, and actigraphy,
    31
Frequency of nocturnal awakenings
    (FNA), 28

Frequency of symptoms, and diagnosis,
    3–4

G
Graphs, of sleep diary data, 49–51,
    63–64, 83–84, 165

H
Headaches, risks and therapy, 20
Health assessment, measurement
    instruments, 27
Home administration, sleep assessment
    measures, 36
Homeostat
    extending sleep opportunity, effects
    of, 39–40
    sleep hygiene information, 71–73
Homeostatic regulation, 14n
Hunger, and sleep, 75
Hyperarousal, 7, 10, 87
    treatment of, 87
Hypnogram, 73
Hypomania, risks and therapy, 20

I
Imagery training, goal of, 19
Indications for therapy, 36–41
Initial insomnia, defined, 2
Insomnia
    behavioral model of, 7–11
    conditioning of and time frame, 40
    and daytime fatigue, 4–5, 5–6
    diagnosis of. See Diagnosis of
    insomnia
    duration of illness, 3–5
    EEG activity, 5
    frequency of symptoms, 3–4
    initial/middle/terminal, 2
    phase-delay component, 20
    primary, 1–2, 22–23
    psychophysiologic insomnia, 2
    secondary, 22
    severity of illness, 3–5
    sleep architectural abnormalities,
    30
    as subjective complaint, 5
    WHO definition, 1, 5
Insomnia Severity Index, 27, 28
    in clinical setting, 35–36

Intake evaluation, 21, 34–48
    assessment algorithm, 37
    contraindications for therapy, 41–43
    goals of, 34–35
    indications for therapy, 36–41
    Insomnia Severity Index, 35–36
    introduction to patient, 35
    medical history form, 166
    medical symptoms checklist, 167
    medication, discontinuing, 45–46
    motivation for change index, 171
    patient questions, 47–48
    patient resistance, 47–48
    setting weekly agenda, 48
    sleep diary, introducing, 46–47
    sleep environment checklist, 170
    symptom checklist, 168–169
    treatment options, presentation of,
        43–44
Intensity of symptoms, and diagnosis,
    4–5
International Classification of Sleep
    Disorders-Revised (ICSD-R),
    definition of insomnia, 2
Internet
    retrospective questionnaires on, 33
    sleep medication certification info, 24

L
Learned sleep-prevention associations,
    meaning of, 2
Light, effects on sleep, 73–74
Lightbox, phototherapy, 19–20

M
Mania
    and insomnia, 42
    risks and therapy, 14, 16, 20
Marijuana use, effects on sleep, 39
Medical conditions
    assessment of, 88
    related to insomnia, 42
Medical history
    information form, 166
    intake information, 27
    medical symptoms, checklist for, 27,
        167
Medications
    common patient questions, 109–113

    for daytime sleepiness, 61–62
    discontinuing, 42, 45–46, 109–113
    for medical conditions, types causing
        insomnia, 42
    and rebound insomnia, 110
    sedative hypnotics, types of, 45
    side effects, 110
    for sleep state misperception, 87
    sleep state on, 109
    as treatment option, 44, 50–51
    withdrawal from, 42, 45, 109–111
    See also Benzodiazepines
Melatonin
    for circadian dysrhythmia, 87
    effects on sleep, 39
Methylphenidate, for daytime
    sleepiness, 61–62
Middle insomnia, defined, 2
Motivation for change index (MFCI),
    171
Multidimensional Pain Inventory
    (MPI), 27
Multi-Factorial Fatigue Inventory
    (MFI), 27

N
Naps
    resting versus sleeping, 106
    short versus long, 81
    sleep hygiene information, 71, 80–81
Narcolepsy, 42
Neurofeedback
    EEG data for, 21
    effectiveness of, 21
Nicotine, effects on sleep, 77
Nightmare disorder, 42
Nocturnal myoclonus, 42
Noise, effects on sleep, 73–74
Noncompliance. See Patient
    nonadherence

O
Obstructive sleep apnea, 30, 42
Over-the-counter sedatives, effects on
    sleep, 39

P
Pain assessment, measurement
    instruments, 27

Panic disorder
   and insomnia, 42
   risk and therapy, 19
Paradoxical intention, 18
Parasomnias
   and insomnia, 42
   risk and therapy, 14, 16
Patient assessment. *See* Diagnosis of
   insomnia; Sleep assessment
Patient compliance, and minimal gains,
   68–70
Patient nonadherence, 64–70
   call in approach to, 84
   cognitive restructuring approach to,
      67, 84
   indicated by sleep diary data, 64,
      83
   patient reasons/clinical responses,
      65–67, 84
   and sleep state misperception, 67
Patient questions/concerns, 105–120
Performance anxiety, risk and therapy,
   19
Perpetuating factors, 8–10
   discussing with patient, 52–55
Phase advance sleep disorders, 42
Phase delay sleep disorders, 42
Phase-delay component, and therapy,
   20
Phase shifts, and actigraphy, 31
Photosensitivity, risks and light therapy,
   20
Phototherapy, 19–20
   for circadian dysrhythmia, 87–88
   contraindications to, 20
   mechanisms of action, 20
   time of day for, 20
Pittsburgh Sleep Diary, example pages,
   172–173
Pittsburgh Sleep Quality Index (PSQI),
   27, 28
Poikilothermia, of REM sleep, 75
Polysomography (PSG), 30–31
   advantages of, 30
   functions of, 30
   measures of, 30
   substance abuse indications, 88
Posttraumatic stress disorder, and
   insomnia, 42

Precipitating factors, 8, 10
   discussing with patient, 52–53
Predisposing factors, 7–8, 10
   discussing with patient, 52–53
Prescribed time to bed (PTIB), 28
Prescribed time out of bed (PTOB), 28
Primary insomnia
   defined, 1–2
   diagnosis of, 23
   as psychophysiologic insomnia, 2
Problem-solving, avoiding at bedtime,
   78–79
Progressive muscle relaxation, goal of,
   19
Prospective measures, 28–29
   purpose of, 28
   sleep diary, 28–29
Psychiatric illness
   assessment of, 27, 88
   as contraindication for therapy, 14,
      16, 20
   related to insomnia, 42
Psychological factors, in insomnia, 8
Psychophysiologic insomnia, definition
   of, 2

Q
Questionnaires, diagnostic, 26–28
   general information measures, 27
   psychiatric instruments, 27

R
Rebound insomnia, and medications,
   110
Relapse prevention, 99–104
   insomnia reoccurrence, actions to
      take, 101–104
   long term versus short term
      prescription, 100
Relaxation training
   contraindications to, 19
   forms of, 19
   for hyperarousal, 87
   information sources on, 19
   practice before use, 19
   for sleep state misperception, 86
REM sleep
   awakenings following, 78
   and thermoregulation, 75

Reports, by clinicians, case example, 121–141
Resistance of patient, 47–48
  motivation for change index, 171
  See also Patient nonadherence
Restless legs syndrome, 30, 42
Retrospective measures, 26–28
  assessment instruments, list of, 27
  purpose of, 26
  See also Sleep assessment
Rituals, disadvantages of, 39
Rumination, and insomnia, 8

S
Schizophrenia, and insomnia, 42
Secondary insomnia, 22
Sedative hypnotics. See Medications
Self-medication, forms of, 39
SF-36 Health Survey, 27
Short sleep, versus insomnia, 5
Sigma activity, substance abuse indications, 88
Situational factors, related to insomnia, 42, 73–74
Sleep
  circadian regulation of, 14n
  homeostatic regulation of, 14n
  normal, duration in hours, 4
  stages of, 78
  thought and cognition during, 65–66
Sleep architectural abnormalities, defined, 30
Sleep assessment, 26–33
  actigraphy, 31–33
  assessment algorithm, 37
  Epworth Sleepiness Scale (ESS), 27
  general information, 27
  health and pain assessment, 27
  home administration, 36
  Insomnia Severity Index, 27, 28, 35–36
  Multi-Factorial Fatigue Inventory (MFFI), 27
  Pittsburgh Sleep Quality Index (PSQI), 27, 28
  polysomography (PSG), 30–31
  prospective measures, 28–29
  psychiatric assessment, 27

retrospective measures, 26–28
sleep diary, 28–29
Sleep compression, 20–21
  goal of, 20
  compared to sleep restriction therapy (SRT), 20
Sleep continuity, defined, 4n
Sleep continuity variables, types of, 28
Sleep deprivation, and daytime fatigue, 4–5
Sleep diary
  common patient questions, 105–109
  functions of, 29
  introducing to patient, 46–47
  nonadherence, indications of, 64, 83
  as prospective measure, 28–29
  review/graphing during treatment, 49–51, 63–64, 83–84, 165
  single page format, 28–29, 172–173
  sleep continuity variables, 28, 46–47
  sleep efficiency (SE measure, 28
  technological aids, 29
  TIB/TST mismatch, interpretation of, 51–52
  tracking variables measured, 28
  Week at a Glance format, 174
Sleep disorder center, location of clinic, 25
Sleep disorders
  circadian dysrhythmia, 87–88
  listing of, 42
  versus medical conditions, 88
  obstructive sleep apnea, 30, 42
  parasomnias, 14, 16, 42
  phase advance sleep disorders, 42
  phase delay sleep disorders, 42
  polysomography (PSG) recording of, 30
  restless legs syndrome, 30, 42
  sleep state misperception, 42, 85–87
  versus substance abuse, 88
  symptom checklist, 168–169
  See also Insomnia
Sleep efficiency (SE measure
  interpretation of, 40
  purpose of, 28
Sleep environment
  checklist for, 27, 170

optimal for sleep, 73–75
poor, causes of, 42
Sleep hygiene education, 70–82
on alcohol use, 76–77
on bedroom environment, 73–75
benefits of, 70–71
on caffeine, 71, 75–76
in combined approach, 17
effectiveness of, 17
on exercise, 73
on forcing sleep, 79–80
on homeostat/wake time, 71–73
instructions to patients, 18, 71–73
on meals/fluid intake, 75–76
on napping, 71, 80–81
on nicotine effects, 77
patient "to-do" list, 71
on problem-solving at bedtime,
78–79
Sleeping pills. See Medications
Sleep latency (SL), 28, 46, 50
Sleep medicine clinic
brochure, example of, 163–164
ideal setting for, 25
office of clinician, 25
in sleep disorder center, 25
Sleep medicine practitioners
credentialing of, 23–24
office of, 25
patient report, example of, 121–141
structuring sessions by. See
Cognitive-behavioral therapy
sessions
training/expertise of, 23–24
Sleep opportunity, extending, effects of,
39–40
Sleep pressure, reduction, effects of,
39–40
Sleep restriction therapy (SRT),14–16
and cognitive-behavioral
therapy,14–15
contraindications to, 16
daytime sleepiness, dealing with,
61–62
effectiveness of, 16
instructions to patients, 15
less than optimal gains, 69
paradoxical effects, 16

patient concerns, 118–120
patient nonadherence, 64–67
setting prescription with patient,
55–59
compared to sleep compression, 20
wake-up time concerns, 15
Sleep state misperception, 42, 85–87
defined, 31
diagnosis of, 31, 85
discussing with patient, 85–86
and nonadherence, 67
treatment of, 86–87
Sleep titration, 63–70, 83–104
cognitive restructuring, 89–96
goals of, 63, 83, 89, 97–98
minimal/no gains, 68–70, 83–84
nonadherence, dealing with, 64–70,
84
reassessment issues, 84–88
relapse prevention, 99–104
sleep diary data review/graphing,
63–64, 83–84, 89, 97–98
treatment gains, review of, 99
Social factors, in insomnia, 8
Somatized tension, meaning of, 2
Stimulant use
caffeine, 71, 75–76
to counter daytime fatigue, 39
Stimulus control theory, 9–11, 13
Stimulus control therapy (SCT),
12–14
behavioral principles of, 13–14
contraindications to, 14
instructions to clients, 12–13
patient concerns, 118–120
setting prescription with patient,
55–59
Stimulus dyscontrol, meaning of, 9
Stress diathesis model, 7–9
predisposing/precipitating/perpetuati
ng factors, 7–9
Subjective criteria, pros/cons of, 5
Substance use, PSG indications for, 87
Symptom checklist, 27, 168–169

T
Temperature of room, and sleep, 74–75
Terminal insomnia, defined, 2

Therapeutic relationship, 24–25
Thermoregulation, and REM sleep, 75
30-minute rule, 37
Thought process, during sleep, 65–66
Time in bed (TIB), 46, 50, 63
Time to bed (TTB), 50
Time out of bed (TOB), 28, 50
"To-do" list, 59–61, 71
Total sleep opportunity (TSO), 68
Total sleep time (TST), 28, 41, 46–47, 50, 63, 83
   minimal gains and future, 101
Tracking variables, types of, 28
Treatment approaches. *See* Cognitive-behavioral therapies
Treatment graphs. *See* Graphs
Treatment initiation, 49–62
   behavioral model, introduction of, 52–55
   daytime sleepiness, addressing, 61–62
   goals of session, 49
   patient "to-do" list, 59–61

sleep diary data review/graphing, 49–52
Sleep Restriction (SR) prescription, 55–59
stimulus control (SC) prescription, 55–59
Treatment options, presenting to patient, 43–44

W
Wake after sleep onset time (WASO), 28, 46, 50
Week at a Glance format, sleep diary, 174
Weekly agenda, setting during intake, 48
Withdrawal, from sedative hypnotics, 42, 45, 109–111
World Health Organization (WHO), definition of insomnia, 1, 5

Z
Zaleplon, 44
Zolpidem, 44